No Sweat! It's Just Menopause

-Eating, Exercise and Essential Oils for a Healthy CHANGE-

Jill Lebofsky

DISCLAIMER- The author is not a doctor. Please consult your medical doctor for any problems, concerns or questions related to your menopause experience. This book is not meant to treat, diagnose or cure anyone. The information shared is based on the author's professional experience, research and personal observations. Products exclusive to Young Living® are trademarked. All product descriptions, usage directions and photographs are the author's. Author is a Young Living Independent Distributor.

This book is dedicated to Larry-My forever love, best friend, partner on this amazing journey called "life" and my editor extraordinaire. He continues to always support my crazy ideas. According to my teen daughter, he may now "know more about menopause than any man on the planet."

TABLE OF CONTENTS

men - o - pause

Menopause. Perimenopause. Not very sexy words for what SHOULD be the prime years of our lives. Say it out loud: Men-o-pause. When you hear the word, do you cringe a bit, knowing it refers to you getting older, despite how young you may feel? Do you get nervous because you've been told to expect the dreaded hot flashes and the end of sexual desire? Are you worried about your latest best friend, that new fat around your middle that won't budge even when you starve yourself and exercise? Have you resigned yourself to "Yes, all of the above" and living out your life in moodiness and discomfort?

I decided from the onset of my first recognizable "changes" to not allow menopause to get the better of me. So began my quest for knowledge, help, and believe it or not, overall wellbeing.

I have an admission: I don't do sick. I don't do pain. No time for that nonsense! But I've never been a big medicine person. Hate the side effects, the taste and I can't swallow pills easily. I was a rare bird in a family in which my grandfather was a pharmacist and doctors were thought of as gods. Although I am grateful for traditional medicine, as it has saved many of my family members' lives, as I entered my teens and twenties I began forging my own alternative health path. I have added and removed many different elements of my wellness routine during my journey, but when it comes to feeling physically and mentally healthy in recent years, my go-to natural health solution has become essential oils. (If not familiar with essential oils Chapter 2 will give you all you need to know.) Essential oils are an easy, inexpensive way for me to care for my body's physical health and emotional wellness. My oils have supported my digestive system and helped make eating fun again. They have played a vital role in keeping these old bones active. They have helped me through some very stressful moments. So why not use these same, proven essential oils to ease me through my menopause?

As a health coach and Pilates instructor with a focus on women's wellness for the past 13 years, and currently a perimenopausal wife and mama of two teens, I have helped hundreds of women manage their weight by teaching them proper nutrition and appropriate exercise. However, when it came to women in perimenopause or postmenopause, I found this balanced approach was by itself not always enough to tackle all the uncomfortable changes to women's bodies that were affecting their weight, their sleep and their emotions. A few years ago, I began recommending essential oils to my clients for supporting a healthy weight, sleeping better and soothing their achy muscles and joints.

These women experienced so much early success with only these few changes that I began to suspect essential oils could help with other side effects of their changing bodies. But it wasn't until I experienced firsthand my own "changes" that my search for relief became a personal crusade.

Before I started using essential oils to cope with my #1 perimenopausal annoyance, night sweats, I'd wake up every night at 4:00am and tear my blanket off as the heat surged from my forehead to my feet. You know what I'm talking about? A nasty pool of sweat had collected on my stomach. I'd turn the fan to full blast and lift my shirt. By 4:02am I'd be shivering, my sweat freezing cold, so I'd turn away from the fan, bundle back up under the blankets and try to pass out before anything else happened, knowing full well this was neither the first nor the last occurrence that night. This overwhelming heat thing was definitely unwelcome, unsettling, and I needed to get rid of it.

So my pursuit for knowledge and help began. First, because I wasn't messing around, I took a certification course called The 3rd Age Woman® geared toward health/fitness professionals, with a focus on proper eating, exercise and self-care for perimenopausal and postmenopausal women. I also began researching essential oils and their effects on hormonal health. I visited online information sources such as pubmed.gov, which is a website focused on scientific studies and research maintained by the United States National Library of Medicine. I read articles and listened to talks given by health professionals who used essential oils with their patients as opposed to traditional treatments. I listened to essential oil users describe their hunt for relief and heard and read amazing online testimonies about lessening or even eliminating women's menopausal problems. The common theme: Essential oil users were reporting fewer hot flashes, libido had returned and they were feeling more emotionally stable. I started to experiment on myself and my friends and duplicated this success. Victory!! I had found my trifecta–eating, exercise and essential oils–that I needed to face this menopause thing head on.

I wrote this book to help you find an easier solution to your menopausal complaints so you too can stop "sweating it out." First, we will cover some basic information about menopause, hormones, and essential oils. Then we'll explore the most common troubles of women going through THE CHANGE and the incredible, natural, chemical-free ways you can soar through what will be the most exciting, empowering years of your life.

Help is on its way!!

Estrogen ° Progesterone ° Testosterone

OH MY!

This isn't necessarily the "fun" chapter, but it is super important to understand what's going on with our bodies during menopause. I thought about using cutesy language to describe the underlying science of menopause and how it all works to make it a breezier read, but you know what? There's just nothing cute about what we are experiencing. I mean, some women DO glide through menopause the way others do pregnancy and childbirth -- and great for them, that's what we all want for ourselves. But for those of us confronting THE BIG CHANGE, who are always finding an excuse to not have sex, whose husbands and kids are never sure if they're in the presence of Angel Mom or Devil Mom, we just want to know WHY this is happening to us, and we want relief NOW. We want to feel like ourselves again. But to do so, it's important to understand what's going on with our bodies during menopause. So here's the (nearly painless) science lesson. No skipping ahead!

According to the Mayo Clinic, menopause is defined as a natural process in which a woman's ovaries start to decrease in estrogen and progesterone production, "causing hormonal fluctuations and changes in menstruation and fertility." Our bodies are basically telling us we aren't supposed to be having any more babies. (Phew! Sounds good to this mom of two teenagers.) Perimenopause is the beginning of the menopause journey and continues until one is in official menopause after not menstruating for 12 consecutive months. Menopause "is actually a 6- to 13-year process, not an event," advises Dr. Christiane Northrup, author of "The Wisdom of Menopause." In the United States, the average age of women entering menopause is 51.

During my health coaching and menopause coaching certification training, I learned that hormones are often referred to as "chemical messengers." Hormones are largely produced within the endocrine system and then released into the bloodstream. Hormones navigate our bodies, transferring their messages to different cells and tissues and announcing it's time to take action. The primary hormones associated with menopause are estrogen, progesterone, and testosterone, although the stress hormone cortisol also plays a role.

Estrogen: The Star of the Show

Although most of us learned in junior high health class that estrogen was, as my teacher called it, the "happy hormone" and "the star of the show," and was produced in the ovaries, that was really all we learned. And that's actually just the start of the truth about estrogen. The ovaries are part of the endocrine system in women. The endocrine system is a network of chemical messengers that includes all of the glands that make hormones: the adrenal glands, thyroid gland, parathyroid gland, pituitary gland, pineal gland, pancreas and the ovaries in women and testicles in males according to the Mayo Clinic. They regulate metabolism, growth and development, tissue function, sexual function, reproduction, sleep and mood. Estrogen is produced mainly in the ovaries, but also in the adrenal glands, the liver, in fat tissue and in the tissues in the breasts. Dr. Sara Gottfried, MD, author of *The Hormone Cure*, teaches that estrogen refers to a "specific group of hormones responsible for over 400 functions in the female body." That's a big job, far beyond the "happy hormone" lesson from health class! During the most fertile part of our monthly cycle, known as ovulation, our bodies increase estrogen production. The increase in estrogen helps us feel sexy and in the mood for baby-making. (My health teacher didn't teach me THAT either, unless that's what the "happy" hormone *actually* meant.) But as we enter menopause, estrogen production slows down and as a result, our sex drive decreases and many of us experience unwelcome weight gain.

Progesterone: Best Supporting Actress

According to Susan Lark, MD, author of *Hormone Revolution,* progesterone is "the yang to estrogen's yin," and "estrogen expands and progesterone contracts." These two hormones play off of one another, seeking harmony and balance. As estrogen claims the role of the leading lady, progesterone takes on the part of best supporting actress. Like estrogen, progesterone is mostly produced in the ovaries, but the brain and peripheral nervous system provide other needed sources of this critical hormone. Progesterone's main purpose is to prepare the body for pregnancy, but as with estrogen, it also helps to increase libido. For menopausal women, if progesterone levels are low, hot flashes may occur and sex drive decreases. Many women also experience "fuzzy" thinking, mood swings and trouble sleeping.

When a woman's estrogen level is low, she may experience some changes similar to those caused by low progesterone as in the hot flashes and night sweats. Libido lessens and vaginal lubrication decreases. The skin's appearance changes, becomes dry and not as supple. Many women experience memory lapses. My mother in law refers to this newfound forgetfulness as her "senior moments." To that I say: Help! I'm not ready!

Estrogen Dominance: Xenoestrogens

Women can also experience an excess of estrogen, referred to as estrogen dominance. Naturopath Amy LaRue, ND, of The Women in Balance Institute, discusses how this extra estrogen can come from all the chemical filled junk we eat, smell and slather on our bodies in the form of food, perfumes and soaps. LaRue teaches that chemical compounds called xenoestrogens, derived from petroleum-based products, "lodge in our fat cells and are not biodegradable," and don't budge without a thorough detoxification of our bodies. These chemical compounds contribute to our stubborn inability to lose the weight that previously came off with regular diet and exercise. These unwanted chemical invaders can sit in our cells for years, wreaking havoc on our health, specifically on our hormonal health. In the 1980's the Environmental Protection Agency (EPA) conducted a program called the National Human Adipose Tissue Survey. They discovered that ALL human fat samples contained traces of four industrial solvents and one dioxin (a chemical contaminant.) Nine more chemicals were found in more than 90% of the samples. These manmade chemical compounds are some of the major culprits behind so many physical and emotional issues women face throughout their entire lives. Xenoestrogens mimic the effects of estrogen in the body, which leads to the creation of more estrogen, which can result in estrogen dominance. These excessive estrogen levels can cause problems ranging from PMS, fibroids, ovarian cysts, and depression to ovarian and breast cancers.

The skin is the largest organ in the body and, while it may come as a surprise to you, everything you rub on your skin absorbs into the body, gaining direct access to your bloodstream. I don't know about you, but I prefer to keep my blood free from petroleum- based chemicals. How do you know whether the personal care products you use every day are a potential source of xenoestrogens? One way is to search the ingredients on virtually every product you use on or in your body. Two reliable sources are the Environmental Working Group at www.ewg.org which includes the Skin Deep® Cosmetics Database and the Think Dirty® app.

While there are several ingredients that should raise the red flag, the main culprit is parabens. Parabens are chemicals used in the production of lotions, deodorants, shampoos and other personal care products. Their purpose is to help to prevent bacteria and extend shelf life which of course benefits the manufacturer, yet in many countries parabens are banned. Why? Parabens are carcinogens. A quick Google search reveals that parabens are found in 99% of all breast tumors. Ninety-nine percent! If that doesn't stop you from rubbing dangerous creams on your skin, I don't know what will. When I found out my favorite cosmetic-counter, high-end skincare line was loaded with parabens, our twenty-plus year relationship ended instantly. Hundreds of dollars in skincare products when out with the trash, but it wasn't the money that hurt the most. I felt betrayed by a company I'd trusted all of my adult life. How dare they expose me to dangerous chemicals to save a buck? To this day, this particular cosmetic line has not changed its ingredients and I cringe when I hear other women talking about running to the department store to get the next "free gift" because it may cost them their lives or at least their health. Be a savvy consumer. Read ingredients carefully and look for products labeled "Paraben-free." As knowledge of the dangers associated with parabens becomes more mainstream, many manufacturers are jumping on the bandwagon and removing parabens from their products. Still, dangerous chemicals could be lurking in your bathroom. Protect yourself and your family and review the ingredients of every personal care product you use. Eliminate anything with butylparaben, methylparaben and propylparaben. Commit to doing the big clean out. Do it today and bring a big garbage bag, because if your bathroom is anything like mine was when I went paraben-free a few years ago, it's going to fill it up quickly. The good news is, after you clean out, you get to replace the dangerous products with new, safer, all-natural alternatives. I'll even show you how to make some fabulous all-natural, safe, cost-effective personal care products later in this book.

As if parabens weren't scary enough, wait, there's more, lurking in your refrigerator and freezer. Another major offender to women's health from these synthetic compounds are found in commercially raised meat and dairy, because they are contaminated with the genetically modified recombinant bovine growth hormone (rBGH or rBST), used to stimulate milk production in cows. These artificial hormones have been banned in many countries since 2000 but not the US. Best to cut down on these products and seek out ones that are hormone-free and grass fed.

Dump your old glass, toilet, counter, and floor cleaners, your dish soaps and laundry detergents. According to the American Lung Association, we should "choose products that do not contain or have reduced amounts of volatile organic compounds (VOC's), fragrance, irritants . . . [And] avoid using air fresheners altogether." Be aware that manufacturers are not obligated by U.S. law to include on the label all the ingredients found in a product. Just because it is a "green" product doesn't automatically mean it is safer, which is exactly why knowing the source of these products is so important. As for alternatives, I trust products from the company Young Living® for reasons covered in the next chapter. Their Thieves® cleaning products such as dish soap and laundry detergent are plant based, chemical free and essential oil infused. The Thieves Household Cleaner® can replace all of those everyday cleaners, and is a quick and easy fix to lessen your exposure to the sprays and powders which I consider to be the #1 contributor to many unwanted menopausal problems.

Would you like some weed killer on your salad? Non-organic salad greens are sprayed with pesticides and herbicides and even if you wash them well, the dangerous chemicals don't go away. They linger in the very cellular structure of high-water fruits and vegetables like lettuce and berries. We are going to be talking about choosing more fresh produce for a healthy menopause. Choose organic, whenever possible. You are worth it!

Hidden in the soft plastics commonly used as packaging material is another major source of these synthetic chemical invaders. Plastic wrapped foods heated in the microwave contain some of the highest chemical levels. Avoid canned goods, which are usually lined with a plastic coating that contains BPA, a known xenoestrogen. Another great reason for whole food eating!

An offender you might not have suspected is disposable menstrual products. If you are still getting your period or have menstruating daughters, take note. The FDA has detected chemical contaminants in commercial tampons that may increase the risk of cancer, reproductive and developmental problems, heart disease and diabetes. Avoid tampons and sanitary napkins that contain chlorine, fragrance, wax and rayon. I've been menstruating since I was 11 years old, which means I've been using feminine products for a long time. I remember my dad joking when my sister and I were teens that he should buy stock in a tampon company with all the women in his household. Not so funny now that we understand what we've been unknowingly doing to our bodies for years.

What about condoms? Many women in perimenopause and post menopause struggle with issues in the bedroom. Could these latex pregnancy and disease preventers also be part of the problem? If you are still fertile, you may want to take a look at this contraceptive method a little closer. Condoms aren't regulated and don't require a detailed list of ingredients. Do a little research and you'll find that condoms contain chemicals like benzocaine and lidocaine, which are local anesthetics meant to delay a man's climax.

Condoms typically come rolled up and can be a pain to unravel, and may even rip in the attempt. To prevent this issue, companies may add a dry dusting powder, made up of who- knows-what, which isn't necessarily listed on the label. And many condom brands include as a preservative an additional ingredient I must mention . . . again. You guessed it. More parabens.

There are two other types of synthetic estrogen to watch for. Equine estrogen is derived from the urine of pregnant horses and used in the hormone treatments doctors regularly prescribe for menopausal symptoms, such as Premarin and Preempak C. YUK! There are also estrogens created in a lab and used in birth control pills to control irregular menstrual cycles and bleeding. DO NOT USE IF YOU ARE POST MENOPAUSAL. These are simply too potent.

Phytoestrogens – The Natural Alternative

The purpose of this book is to share how essential oils can be used as natural alternatives to support your perimenopause and postmenopause. Some essential oils are phytoestrogens, which The Merriam-Webster dictionary defines as a chemical compound that occurs naturally in plants and has estrogenic (relating to, caused by or being an estrogen) properties. We get most of our phytoestrogens from food. An article from 2011 in *Pharmacognosy Reviews* mentions that estrogenic herbs have been used in the treatment of menopausal symptoms for several thousand years in Asian countries. Other recent studies may help identify potential health benefits and the ability of phytoestrogens to protect against certain diseases. Studies by both Aldercreutz and Mazur and by Messina et al. suggest phytoestrogens act "as cancer prevention and as treatment for menopausal symptoms and osteoporosis." Osteoporosis, a condition in which the bones become weak and brittle, is a serious issue faced by menopausal women. Weight bearing exercises can also help to combat osteoporosis, which we will cover in a later chapter. When precise extraction and distillation processes are used to keep the purity levels and benefits of the oil intact (as Young Living® does), essential oils taken from these plants can provide a natural source of phytoestrogens.

According to a study out of Tulane University, "many plants produce chemicals that mimic or interact with hormone signals in animals." Phytoestrogens bind to estrogen receptors and act in similar ways to estrogen produced naturally in the body. They can also effectively block other more harmful estrogens from binding to estrogen receptors. The Tulane study reports, "Phytoestrogens are weaker estrogens than naturally produced estrogen and the potent synthetic estrogens used in birth control pills."

Since the ovarian production of estrogen and progesterone decreases during menopause, the secondary sources of production of these hormones become important. If your body produces the optimal level of these hormones, then there should be a balance between estrogen and progesterone and you should be virtually free of menopausal problems. Yes, you read that right: PROBLEM FREE!!

Testosterone

According to the North American Menopause Society, testosterone is referred to as the "male" hormone, but it also plays a key role in women's sexual health. Testosterone is produced in the ovaries which continue to produce it even after estrogen production stops. Testosterone levels contribute to libido and may help maintain one's bone and muscle mass, both of which can decrease with age. Testosterone levels do decrease over time, not due to menopause but as a natural result of aging; testosterone levels in women may have already decreased by 50% by the time menopause begins. Testosterone also influences one's stamina levels and the ability to achieve restful sleep, two areas affected during menopause.

Cortisol

Another important hormone that impacts menopause is cortisol, which is produced in the adrenal glands. As mentioned earlier, the adrenal glands are part of the endocrine system which includes the ovaries, and are a secondary source of estrogen and progesterone production. The adrenal glands contribute nearly 50% of postmenopausal hormones during menopause, as the ovaries slow their contribution to hormone production. Dr. Andrew Neville, naturopathic doctor and adrenal specialist, writes that the "ovarian and adrenal hormones are intimately connected." When you are chronically overworked, physically and mentally exhausted, emotionally stressed, you overtax the hormone production of your adrenal glands, and you deplete a large part of your energy. You may experience problems falling asleep and staying asleep and then have to drag yourself out of bed each morning. Food cravings increase along with the need for more sugar and salt. If you have adrenal fatigue, you feel tired even when you do get a good night's sleep.

Ideally, your adrenal glands will produce adequate estrogen to make up for slowed ovarian hormone production during menopause.

The "fight or flight" response that occurs due to a perceived harmful event, attack or threat to survival is triggered by stress and activates those organs needed for survival, such as the heart and lungs, and causes organs less vital to immediate survival to rest and relax, such as the reproductive system and thyroid. The stress response at its most extreme may completely shut off all estrogen, progesterone and testosterone production in your body.

Ann Louise Gittleman, best-selling author of more than 30 books including *Before the Change: Taking Charge of Your Perimenopause*, writes, "Stress increases the levels of cortisol which contributes to estrogen dominance." Gittleman continues, "Cortisol also causes us to retain tummy fat." Ann Louise isn't referring to the easy fat that disappears after a few healthy meals or a nighttime walk. She means the kind of fat that likes to stick around and settle in for the long term. Increased cortisol levels also increase insulin levels, which cause your blood sugar to drop so that you crave sugary, fatty foods. This can be a major contributor to those new pounds. Shawn W. Talbott, PhD, a nutritional biochemist, defines the bottom line as

"More stress = more cortisol = more junk food cravings = more belly fat"

When the adrenals are overstressed or stressed for long periods, they crash and need assistance with functioning. Progesterone is the raw material for cortisol. According to the National Integrated Health Associates website, "When the adrenals are exhausted, the body diverts progesterone to them to help increase cortisol production, and this reduced progesterone may create estrogen dominance." At the same time, "Excessive cortisol also blocks progesterone receptors, creating even lower progesterone levels and an excess of estrogen."

You can see there are many biological and hormonal factors affecting how one experiences menopause. The best thing you can do for yourself is figure out how to get your body's levels to reach the perfect ebb and flow, allowing you to enjoy these empowering years.

Have you had any hormone testing done? Not a bad place to start to understand what your body needs.

You made it! Thanks for sticking with the science lesson!

NOTES

The Ins & Outs Of Essential Oils

I've referred to essential oils a few times now, but I realize you may have never even heard of essential oils. Or you may already be an avid oiler. Regardless of your experience level, it is important to educate yourself before introducing anything new to your body.

Essential oils can be a great solution to so many of our needs as women, especially as menopausal women. When you finish this book I want you to feel completely comfortable in your understanding of why certain essential oils (along with healthy eating and proper exercise) can be safely and effectively used to support your overall wellness, including during perimenopause and menopause, and how they can replace harmful common products that are contributing to many of the unwelcome issues of menopause.

I believe that when we understand WHY we should do something it becomes easier to consistently take necessary actions. Essential oils aren't one-time fixes, but by including them in your daily wellness routine and eliminating as much exposure as you can to toxins, you can age gracefully, stay in shape and find emotional peace!

Mini Essential Oils 101

So what exactly is an essential oil? The *Essential Oil Desk Reference* defines essential oils as "aromatic, volatile liquids distilled from shrubs, flowers, trees, roots, bushes and seeds." Some essential oils can be found on the outside surface of certain plants. Other essential oils are stored inside the plant, in its leaves or within its seeds. Essential oils are complex, made up of hundreds of chemical compounds. They are highly concentrated thanks to their distillation process (in which the oils are purified by heating or cooling) and are much more potent than dried herbs. The "essence" of the plant's fragrance is what makes it "essential." Centuries ago, what we now call essential oils were called "quintessential oils," named after the fifth element of matter, the ***quintessence*** referring to spirit or life force. (Fun fact: The other four elements are fire, air, earth and water.) Not all plants and flowers produce essential oils. The oils aren't "essential" for the plant's survival, but they are still highly beneficial to the plant's ability to adapt to and thrive in its environment.

Plants, flowers and trees have long been sought after for their natural properties. These properties include rare and powerful extracts and essences that are useful for physical and emotional healing, cooking, and beauty enhancement in addition to their use in spiritual practices. Many people are familiar with essential oils, such as, lavender, peppermint and lemon, but there are literally hundreds more, that, when used correctly, can have powerful positive impact on your health and well-being.

- At least 12 different essential oils are mentioned hundreds of times in the Bible. Proverbs 21:20 says, "There is oil in the house of the wise."
- Cleopatra is said to have practiced beauty regimens that combined flowers, herbs and oils.

- By the 1800's, doctors in England, Germany and France were prescribing essential oils for a variety of illnesses and diseases.
- The term "aromatherapie" was coined in 1928 by French chemist Rene-Maurice Gattefosse who invented the word after he suffered a bad burn and effectively treated himself with essential oils; he later began researching the usage of plants' healing qualities.
- During World War I, French surgeon Jean Valnet used essential oils as antiseptics and wrote the book *The Practice of Aromatherapy.*

A-RO-MA-THER-A-PY

noun

Inhalation or bodily application (as by massage) of fragrant essential oils (as from flowers and fruits) for therapeutic purposes; broadly: the use of aroma to enhance a feeling of well-being

Essential oils have enjoyed a resurgence of popularity in recent years as more health-conscious people seek alternatives to traditional Western medicine and learn about natural solutions for looking and feeling their best.

Essential Oils: Their Role in Plants

Some essential oils have therapeutic value, and others are used only for fragrance. Of the more than 300,000 known plant types that exist on earth (with new species being discovered all the time), only 400 to 500 produce essential oils. Essential oils play a significant biological role within plants. According to an article found on the National Association for Holistic Aromatherapy's (NAHA) website, essential oils' ultimate purpose is to "help the plant to adapt to the ever-changing internal and external environment.

Recent scientific research has shown that plants produce essential oils for a variety of purposes." The three main parts oils play in a plant's welfare are *The Attractor, The Defender and The Healer.* Oils can play a similar role in our bodies.

The Attractor – Bees, butterflies, small birds and other insects are drawn to the plant's aromatic release which helps ensure cross pollination, just as we use perfume to attract a mate.

The Defender – The plant's oil can help it put up a good fight and defend itself from animals and insects, and against competing plants from invading its turf. You can use those same oils to defend yourself in many different ways, the least of which is to scare off those same annoying bugs that buzz around us on a hot summer evening (one less thing for *this* hormonal mama to be annoyed with).

The Healer – According to the NAHA website, the oils "protect the plant by their antifungal and antibacterial nature" and act "against a wide range of organisms that may threaten the survival of the plants." Did you know that modern day prescription medicines are botanically-based? Essential oils act as nature's built-in recipes for wellness. Do some of your own research about these essential oils and how they can support your body in a zillion different ways.

Not All Oils Are Created Equal

When we use essential oils to support and create balance in our bodies, making sure we use the highest quality of oil is, well, essential! We want our oils to do what they are meant to—help us gain control of our moods, increase our energy levels and make our bodies feel great. Unfortunately, as more people learn about and seek the benefits of essential oils, new consumers are exposed to tons of inferior, copycat products hitting the market as companies cash in on the growing demand. These products are packaged up all pretty, given whimsical names, and oftentimes they are virtually indistinguishable from true, pure essential oils. As exciting as it is to see people turning to essential oils instead of turning to the pharmacy counter, the new reality is that my local drugstore now sells oils! Oils are suddenly everywhere, and the companies producing and marketing them are counting on the consumer's lack of knowledge. Unfortunately, most people (not you—you and I know better or are about to!) aren't educated about the difference between unadulterated essential oils and what's being mass marketed on retail shelves and on sites like Amazon®. Your drugstore cashier, heck even your pharmacist likely hasn't researched oils to know there are critical quality differences between brands. If you intend to use an essential oil for a specific purpose, and if you want it to do what it's supposed to, then you should consider the source of the oil, including whether it comes from a non-GMO seed (not genetically engineered), and whether the oil is cultivated without using pesticides. You owe it to yourself and to your body to learn the facts and not simply assume that clever but meaningless marketing words such as "pure" and "natural" mean your oil hasn't been tampered with. Has the oil you're considering using even been extracted from the plant in such a way to preserve its benefits? The specific method of getting the oil out of the plant may not seem like a big deal, but if you want it to work, it can mean everything! You should inquire whether the oils you're purchasing are distilled without alcohol or chemical solvents or additives, as most oils on the market are processed through these non-natural means. If someone can't answer these questions, then dig deeper and do some research to find the answers before you put the oil in or on your body.

I personally don't want to worry about where my oil comes from. I did my research— exhaustively. I compared brands and read everything I could find. Based on my findings, I choose to buy Young Living® essential oil products exclusively due to the high standards of their Seed to Seal Promise® and close attention to sourcing, science and standards.

With Young Living® oils, all you get in the bottle is what the label says. For more information on the farming, cultivation process and science behind Young Living® essential oils, visit www.seedtoseal.com. For the purposes of this book, I will only be referring to Young Living® essential oils and their oil infused products.

Three Ways To Gain The Benefits of Essential Oils

There are three ways to bring the benefits of essential oils into your body: topically, through inhalation, and by ingestion. Some oils have one method of use, whereas some have two or three. When using essential oils to support positive hormonal changes in your life, you will experience maximum results if you use them in all three ways, but if you're not comfortable with one, you can absolutely get great results from the other methods.

Inhalation

As a child I was enthralled with the life of Helen Keller. She had to rely on her sense of touch, taste and smell to experience the world. I love her quote, "Smell is a potent wizard that transports us across thousands of miles and all the years we have lived."

Inhaling oils is the most common way people experience essential oils and where most people start. Nothing could be easier. Open the bottle and place it under your nose, or put a drop in your palms, rub hands together, cup nose and inhale. Inhaling an oil such as Peppermint may help one get rid of the yucky feeling one gets after overeating. Breathing in Lavender may support your respiratory system and help you get a good night's sleep.

Many people use a cold air diffuser to inhale their oils. It is a safer alternative to scented candles, air fresheners and incense, all which emit carcinogens into the air which often linger for weeks. A few drops of essential oils are placed in the diffuser which mixes the oils with the water in its tank. The diffuser lets out a fine mist to infuse the air in the room with a beautiful aroma that has therapeutic benefits for everyone in your home.

When inhaled, essential oils affect the emotional center of your brain, called the limbic system, within approximately 20 to 30 seconds. In the book *Aromatherapy: A-Z*, Higley and Higley state, "The limbic system is directly connected to those parts of the brain that control heart rate, blood pressure, breathing, memory, stress levels and hormone balance." This explains why smells often bring up memories or emotions and why aromatherapy can have, in addition to physiological benefits, such profound psychological benefits. Have you ever smelled freshly baked bread and were transported back to grandma's kitchen, or smelled cologne on a passerby that instantly had you thinking of your high school boyfriend?

Your brain and your reproductive system are closely connected. If you've been pregnant, you probably remember how your moods changed without warning or reason and your ability to remember things seemed to come and go? Many women experience similar issues during menopause. Inhaling essential oils is a quick fix for these menopause memory lapses, releasing stress, managing the rollercoaster of emotions and resetting our mood.

One more—and my personal favorite—inhalation method is diffuser jewelry! I put a drop of oil on a lava bead diffuser bracelet before I leave the house, so my oils are always with me for a quick pick-me-up. (Admittedly, I do sniff my wrist a lot!) Any porous substance, from unfinished pottery and wood to cotton and cork, can be used as a diffuser. How easy is that?!

Topical

We've already talked about how substances are absorbed through the skin. Essential oils can be applied topically to the neck, wrists or feet to distribute through the body, or else to a specific body part you're trying to affect. Essential oils are highly concentrated, so only a couple of drops are needed. When applying essential oils directly to the skin, "less is more" is a good beginner's motto until you're experienced enough to understand the degree to which the oils effect you. Those new to essential oils should dilute them to slow the rate of absorption. You can combine essential oils with a carrier oil, which is any fat-based oil such as coconut, grapeseed or jojoba. Carrier oils serve a few purposes: 1) They dilute the oils to avoid sensitivities; 2) They allow the essential oils to spread over a large area (essential oils are absorbed quickly into the skin); and 3) They help use less amount of essential oils allowing your bottles to last longer.

When using essential oils, specifically for menopausal support, you can apply your oils to your inner thigh or inner thigh crease and just below the navel as well as around the ankles. Whoa, wait a sec...Why ankles? Because in the ancient practice of Reflexology, the outer part of the ankle represents the ovaries and the inside part of the ankle represents the uterus and pelvic muscles. Reflexologists believe that applying pressure to specific areas of the feet, hands and ears that correspond to specific body parts and organs will have a direct effect on the body's health.

When in doubt, don't get hung up on WHERE your oils should go, just put them on anywhere (just avoid the eyes and inside of ears and nose). These are smart oils!

Ingestion

I love to take my oils internally, but some people have concerns about ingesting (eating or drinking) oils. MOST oils out there are NOT safe for ingestion. Young Living® is different. They have an entire line of oils called Vitality® that is generally recognized as safe (GRAS) by the Food and Drug Administration. Vitality® oils are what I'm referring to throughout the book whenever I refer to ingesting the oils. That said, the way you use your oils is based entirely on personal preference. If you don't want to ingest them, then don't. The ingestion of oils directly into your mouth, either by putting them into empty vegetable capsules (you can purchase online or at the health food store) or by adding them as an ingredient in a food or a beverage, are simply additional and effective ways of getting essential oils into your body. If you choose to ingest your oils, it is 100% critical to first read the label and to know the source of your oil. If a product label claims you're holding a bottle of "pure" or "natural" essential oil, but the bottle's warning says you can't ingest it, then you must question its purity. Although, there are some essential oils that are never safe internally no matter the source, this is why education is so important.

Even though Young Living Vitality® oils are perfectly safe to ingest, you should pace yourself. As with introducing any new food into your body, you should begin everything in moderation. There's no hurry or need to overdo it, as you will quickly learn what feels right for your body. Some people like to add a few drops of oils to their water or to their morning smoothies for weight management and for a workday energy boost. Cooking with essential oils is a great way to enhance the flavor of certain meals (a single drop of lemon oil can provide the same flavor as half a squeezed lemon) and to get the benefit of the oil. If you do ingest your oils, it is important to use your oils only in glass, ceramic or stainless steel containers. Many a favorite plastic cup or water bottle has been ruined by oils that break down the toxins in the plastic, and since those toxins have nowhere else to go except into your beverage, I repeat: Use in glass, ceramic or stainless steel containers only. Check out my rules of thumb at the end of this chapter before cooking with oils. It will save you some ruined meals.

Oils are easy. There are many ways to enjoy them, and no excuse to be without!

COOKING WITH ESSENTIAL OILS RULES OF THUMB

There may be 60 drops in a teaspoon if you measure, but you will most definitely ruin your dish if you use a teaspoon of essential oils, and it will most likely not be good for you. Here are some helpful hints for utilizing essential oils in the best way.

1) Don't drip your oils right into the food. Drip them onto a separate spoon. Rarely does just one drop come out of the bottle, and 2 drops could overpower your dish.

2) If a recipe calls for one teaspoon of citrus juice, use 1 drop of oil to start, taste, and add another if needed.

3) If it calls for one tablespoon of citrus oil start with 3-4 drops and add to taste.

4) Add 4-6 drops to replace the zest of fresh fruit and slowly add more if wanted.

5) If recipe calls for one teaspoon or less of a stronger flavored herb or spice such as oregano, basil, rosemary, thyme, sage, dill, black pepper, cinnamon bark, clove, ginger, nutmeg, thieves or peppermint, use the toothpick method. Dip a toothpick in the essential oil and then swirl it into the recipe to blend with the other ingredients.

   Don't put toothpick back into bottle. If you want more use the other end or a new toothpick!

6) If using oils to flavor water you MUST use glass, stainless steel or ceramic, not plastic cups.

   The oils will pull the toxins from the plastic into the liquid. If you are putting them into a smoothie, the oils will be more diluted and mixed in so it is OK in a plastic cup, but don't let it sit there for a long time and be sure to wash out the cup when finished.

7) Use organic ingredients. This may not always possible due to lack of access to organic foods where you live or the cost, but do so when possible. The oils are supporting a gentle detoxification of your body, so it makes no sense to add toxins back in. FYI Young Living® makes an all-natural, toxin free fruit & veggie wash infused with Thieves® oil. It's great to have on hand!

8) When heated, essential oils will lose their potency. That is why it is best to add oils at the end of a recipe after removing from heat when possible or at the end of the boiling, baking or simmering process.

NOTES

One Hot Mama

All right now! Let's get started with what you have been patiently waiting for: natural solutions! Let's begin with some common issues among perimenopausal women: hot flashes and night sweats. According to Johns Hopkins Medicine Health Library, *Introduction To Menopause,* " Hot flashes or flushes are, by far, the most common symptom of menopause, with about 75% of all women experiencing sudden, brief, periodic increases in their body temperature." Those episodes may include the night sweats, which often make sleeping patterns more erratic, something I can personally vouch for. Remember my old sweat/freeze all night routine? Are your nights similar? Perhaps. Inevitable? No way!

Hot Flashes

Hot Flashes or Flushes are caused by (get ready for a mouthful) vasomotor instability. Dr. Mark Smith, Jr., wrote an article for obgyn.net that illustrates this phenomenon perfectly. First, you need to understand that blood vessels can widen or narrow depending upon what the body tells them to do. If the body gets hot, then it sends blood to the surface by widening the blood vessels to allow the heat to leave the body. The body has a built-in regulatory mechanism for heat control, and a thermoregulator in the brain acts as the body's thermostat. The thermoregulator in a woman's brain controls her body's heat and cooling just as the thermostat in her house controls the heater and air conditioner.

Imagine someone is constantly moving the thermostat up and down (ironically, this is a reality in most menopausal households as no one agrees on what the *true* temperature is), causing the air conditioner to repeatedly start and stop. Hot flashes are a woman's thermostat bouncing up and down. Seemingly out of nowhere, the thermoregulator tells her body it is hot. It sends blood rushing to the skin's surface causing a flush or redness. Then the body tries to cool itself by sweating. Eventually the thermostat resets itself.

These surges can come on at any time and may pass quickly, but they can also last up to a half an hour. One thing's for sure: They are dreadful! Hot flashes and their partner in crime, the night sweats, may be caused by different factors, but a primary culprit is low progesterone levels.

Dr. Northup writes, "Women with low progesterone but normal estrogen levels may experience hot flashes and night sweats." She also proposes that hot flashes occur with "low testosterone levels" and "increased cortisol." She notes that even "low levels of antioxidants in the body can contribute to hot flashes," which is one reason why a whole food, plant enriched diet is important during the menopausal years. We will discuss how this works in a bit.

Progessence Plus®

Dr. Dan Purser, MD, a doctor specializing in hormones and preventative medicine, has written several books on wellness and disease prevention issues, including one on progesterone. At the Young Living International Grand Convention of 2010 in Salt Lake City, he tested the progesterone levels of thousands of women, and found that 99% of his subjects had effectively zero levels (<0.20 ng/ml) of progesterone in their blood – no matter what their age. This led him to create the Progessence Plus® oil blend for Young Living. According to Dr. Purser, Progessence Plus® "is what we call a highly micronized bio-identical (human) progesterone, in that it has a natural Vitamin E base with a set of special essential oils that include frankincense, copaiba, sandalwood, peppermint and bergamot— that enhance absorption through the skin and also have a calming benefit."

Micronized progesterone helps increase absorption because of its extremely small particles. Progessence Plus® uses wild yam as its source of micronized progesterone. (It can also be made from soy) The wild yam, through the natural compounding process that Young Living® uses, becomes identical in molecular structure to human-produced progesterone.

Regular users of Progessence Plus® have reported their hot flashes and night sweats decreased, that their energy returned and their libido and mood improved.

Place a drop of Progessence Plus® on either side of your neck and around your ankles or on forearms once a day as a great starting point. Monitor how you feel and add another drop to reach the desired benefit, most women find they need just 1 drop once or twice a day so start there. Other women do use a drop when having a hot flash but that can also be too much for some. It's a good idea to pay extra attention to the changes in your body when you start using essential oils. Changes may be subtle and oftentimes once we feel better, we forget how badly we once felt. Keeping track of your progress with a diary of any changes you experience when you incorporate Progessence Plus® into your daily regimen can help you recognize how it is supporting you. For more information directly from Dr. Purser, go to http://bit.ly/2BbpnpX

Clary Sage

Low estrogen is another culprit behind hot flashes and night sweats. Clary Sage essential oil is another great choice for dealing with these menopausal nuisances. Clary Sage is an example of a phytoestrogen, or plant-based estrogen that we discussed in the previous chapter. According to Franchomme & Pénöel (1990), Clary Sage oil is estrogen-like, due to its content of sclareol, which is said to be structurally similar to human estrogen. Used consistently, a drop on the forearms and a drop rubbed in over the lower abdomen, which is directly over the ovaries, 2-3 times a day may contribute to fewer inconvenient hot and sweaty moments. It may improve women's mood, provide support for natural vaginal lubrication and increase libido, related issues which we will discuss in upcoming chapters.

IMPORTANT: It is recommended that, if you are going through perimenopause and it hasn't been a full year since your last period, to be careful with Clary Sage because it may increase fertility. I will not be held responsible for any unintended pregnancies!

Fight Or Flight

Dr. Neville, the adrenal specialist referred to earlier, mentions adrenal glands, adrenal fatigue and low levels of cortisol as possible contributors to hot flashes. We previously discussed how, similar to your ovaries, your adrenal glands produce every ovarian hormone, including progesterone, testosterone and estrogen. As you age, the estrogen production in your ovaries slows, and the adrenal glands become very important in supporting your hormonal health through the menopausal years.

According to Dr. Neville, "in Western cultures, a miserable journey through menopause is common." Why? Because if the adrenal glands are constantly triggered by stress—if you're in "fight-or-flight" mode all the time—it affects your ovarian hormones. Some stress is healthy, even critical for survival, but too much stress is bad for women's hormonal balance during menopause. The adrenal glands produce the stress hormone Cortisol, which is meant to be released during heightened stress and then returned to normal levels after the stressful conditions have passed. It's important to remember that in today's chaotic society, most of us live with heightened stress all the time. We haven't figured out how to turn ourselves off from the stressful stimuli of work, of social media, or the 24 x 7 news cycle. As a result, we experience excess cortisol production which can lead to sleep disturbances and weight gain. In addition, the overproduction of cortisol lowers sex hormone levels and can produce hot flashes. Therefore, the more optimally your adrenal function is working entering this hormonal change of life, the easier your experience should be with the hot flashes. Less optimal adrenal gland function equals more menopausal problems and a much tougher time of it.

Dr. Neville reports that the women in his practice with adrenal fatigue "tend to go through menopause earlier and have more significant symptoms than women whose adrenal function is optimal." He continues, "Women who experience symptoms of menopause are many more times likely to be dealing with adrenal fatigue than women who sail through it symptom-free." If we are to heed Dr. Neville's warning, we should start by addressing the adrenal glands first to reduce adrenal fatigue. You may find that many symptoms disappear when the adrenal glands return to optimal functioning.

Endoflex®

We will cover ways to reduce the toll on your adrenal glands through relaxation and letting go from life's worries in an upcoming chapter. I didn't realize the degree to which stress was affecting my adrenal glands until I added Endoflex® essential oil into my perimenopausal oil regimen, and within a month the frequency of my night sweats and hot flashes had dramatically lessened. Some days and nights, completely sweat free! So much so that I could even wear a sweatshirt to bed and not wake up sweating.

Endoflex® is an essential oil blend which may support the adrenal glands as well as the thyroid. Endoflex® supports a healthy metabolism (an important factor in weight management), can contribute to hormonal balance and has been reported by users to make a woman's hot flashes a thing of the past. Endoflex® users also describe feeling a boost in energy and feeling less stressed out. Endoflex® can be applied to the front of the neck, lower back and feet several times a day and is most effective when used consistently.

Other Essential Oils For Hot Flashes/Night Sweats

Other essential oils that may help you get through the day without dripping in sweat include Geranium, Lemon, Roman Chamomile and Fennel and the Young Living® blends Lady Sclareol® and Sclaressence®, both of which contain Clary Sage oil. Keep a small spray bottle with a few drops of Peppermint essential oil in water in your purse for when your next menopausal "power surge" hits. The Peppermint almost immediately cools the skin's surface. Ahhhh . . . Only use it during the day because the Peppermint oil can be energizing. If you get overheated at night, I have a different spray you can try that has a few drops of Peppermint, but mostly Clary Sage, Lavender and the Peace and Calming® essential oil blend which contains Roman Chamomile, which can help you get a good night's sleep. This mix is not quite as cooling as only Peppermint oil, but it usually does the trick without keeping me awake in the process.

Young Living® also makes a body cream called Prenolone Plus® that contains Ylang Ylang, Clary Sage and DHEA. According to the Mayo Clinic, DHEA is a naturally produced hormone in the adrenal gland. "In turn, DHEA helps produce other hormones, including testosterone and estrogen" which can help support our hormonal balance.

Whenever you hear jokes about women and menopause, they usually involve hot flashes. But for those who have experienced hot flashes and night sweats, we know they're no joke. Before going the traditional route, try essential oils. They will need to be applied consistently, and it may take some time to feel the results as your body returns to hormonal balance. But give it a shot!

POWERSURGE PROTECTOR

(for perimenopausal support)

1-2 drop of Progessence Plus® applied to sides of neck and ankles

1-2 drops of Clary Sage applied to forearms and below navel and ankles

1 drop of Endoflex® down front of neck

Apply twice daily.

* use oils with a couple of teaspoons of a carrier oil such as coconut or grapeseed oil if you experience any skin sensitivity

* For on-the-go convenience, put 10-12 drops of each oil into a 10 ml rollerball roll-on and top off with a carrier oil.

"YOU'RE STILL COOL" SPRAY

15-30 drops of Peppermint oil (experiment on yourself)

1/2 tsp. witch hazel

Fill a 4 oz. spray bottle with distilled water ¾ full.

Add in the essential oils, and witch hazel for daytime use.

* At night, use 1 drop of Peppermint, 5 drops of Lavender, 4 drops of Peace & Calming®, 1 drop of Clary Sage, witch hazel and distilled water. If the Peppermint keeps you awake, try eliminating it from the mix.

NOTES

Scentsational Sex

A poll I read in a *Cosmopolitan Magazine Sex and Social Media Survey* from August 15, 2011—yes I know, not very scientific—showed that 1 in 5 women prefer Facebook to sex and 57% would rather give up sex than stop using the internet. Now I love a little scrolling as much as the next gal, but virtual connection over human contact—that's just wrong! This is a time when divorce is becoming less common for younger adults, according to Pew Research Center, and so-called "gray divorce" is on the rise, almost doubling since the 1990's. In "The Epidemic of Gray Divorces," *Psychology Today* reports, "Gray divorce is the term used to refer to those who divorce after age fifty. Some researchers call it a divorce revolution. And the numbers are growing while divorce rates of other age groups are falling."

Jessica O'Reilly, author of *The New Sex Bible,* writes, "Hormonal changes that arise with age can cause significant shifts in sex drive. And though every couple of every age experiences differentials in desire, these can become more pronounced with age." These hormonal changes occurring in women in perimenopause and postmenopause often result in not only to a lack of sexual desire, but the awkwardness of the subject can also lead to a lack of communication of these changes to their partner. Instead of a passionate Saturday night, it's another evening of watching Netflix until you both fall asleep. Lack of communication between couples leads to miscommunication. A week without physical connection turns into a month and even into years. For some it ends in divorce. For single women going through menopause, this lack of libido makes it difficult to make the effort to attract a desired relationship. All because people don't talk about what is happening (or not happening) between the sheets, at least not completely and honestly with anyone, even their best friends. I myself am a TMI (too much information) girl when it comes to talking sex so have no fear, we ARE going there!

The two main complaints about sex at this stage in life are lack of libido and painful intercourse, usually due to vaginal dryness. We learned in Chapter 2 how fluctuating estrogen, progesterone and testosterone levels can lead to a lack of sexual appetite. No one in a loving relationship wants to keep putting off their lover's advances, but putting aside the menopausal lack of sleep, irritability and newfound pounds that leave us feeling less then desirable, these hormones are messing with us and preventing us from getting down and dirty.

I have been in a sexual relationship with my husband for a quarter century. We love and respect each other and are still hot for one another all these years later. But who are we kidding? Our sex life over the past 25 years has had its highs and its lulls. Since we introduced essential oils into the bedroom a few years ago, our intimacy has climbed to a whole new fun level. The oils help me get in the mood after a long, stressful day. They help me to shut off my laundry list of to-do's in my head and enjoy being in the moment with the man I love. They have helped moisten, as one of my clients put it, the "Sahara Desert" between my legs so that all parts glide easily and comfortably. They have also helped my man feel like a man by ensuring everything functions to top performance. Bottom line: Essential oils should be on your night table, close at hand.

Essential oils have been used for sensuality and romance throughout the ages. Sensual images related to scents and fragrances can be seen in the sensual images created by ancient Egyptian writers and artists. The Song of Solomon in the Bible makes references to scents, perfumes and anointing oils. One line says, *"His cheeks are like a bed of spices, banks of scented herbs, his lips are lilies dripping liquid myrrh."* The ancient Hindu text the *Kama Sutra*, AKA the "Bible of Sexuality," refers to aromatherapy.

Decreased levels of progesterone or estrogen during menopause can lead to decreased feeling of sexual desire. The same oils used for hot flashes in the previous chapter can be used to support a healthy libido. Progessence Plus® and Clary Sage help support your body's hormones and in doing so naturally increase your sexual wants and needs.

Other essential oils can play a central role in supporting and boosting a menopausal woman's sex life. Let's face it: At this point in our lives, we need some warming up. We need to feel sexy and romantic to get the party started. Sexual excitement can start with the nose. The best place to start is to diffuse oils in the bedroom. When you inhale an essential oil it goes through to your limbic system, which is in charge of your emotions. Within just a few minutes, whatever annoys you about your mate doesn't seem so bad; instead, he's looking darn good with his unshaved salt and pepper scruff. This is partially due to the oils stimulating the pituitary gland which controls your hormones. Not only are the oils directly influencing your mood, but they are improving your hormonal health, which in turn can affect your libido.

Ylang Ylang

The scent of both Ylang Ylang and Jasmine essential oils is intoxicating. Both oils are found in the blends Joy® and Sensation®. Remember how one of the things the oil of the plant does is release a scent to attract insects for cross-pollination to help the plant reproduce? Well, Ylang Ylang has been a powerful attractor of the opposite sex and an aphrodisiac since ancient times. It may promote sexual energy and balance between the sexes, may intensify eroticism and is good to help you release your inhibitions and try some experimenting between the sheets.

Jasmine

Jasmine has long been used in the act of seduction, romance and attraction. It may boost confidence or elevate your sexual awareness. Jasmine may also relieve stress, remove emotional blocks and calm anxiety before sex.

Joy®

The oil blend Joy® combines Ylang Ylang, Jasmine, Rose and other sensual essential oils. Rose oil is always associated with love and romance.

Sensation®

The Sensation® blend is similar to Joy®, but its combination of oils applied on those sweet spots (see below) makes you feel all tingly! It is also used in Sensation Body Lotion® and in Sensation Massage Oil®.

Neroli

Neroli oil is derived from orange blossoms. Findings in a randomized controlled trial by Choi, SY, Kang, P, Lee HS, Seol GH, "indicate that inhalation of Neroli oil helps relieve menopausal symptoms, increase sexual desires and reduce blood pressure in post- menopausal women." Neroli oil may help unlock your passion and increase sensitivity to your partner's touch. It has a calming, as well as an aphrodisiac, effect. Great for date night!

Application

In addition to diffusing, topical use of essential oils can help bring back that loving feeling. The best place to apply these oils is on or in the crease of the inner thigh or below the navel. Because the scent draws your partner in close, a drop on the breasts or neck never hurts. If you choose to place the oils in sensitive areas, test them first on your forearm to see how they feel. Should you have any problem after putting them on more sensitive places, grab a carrier oil and dilute—don't jump in the shower. Oils and water do not mix!

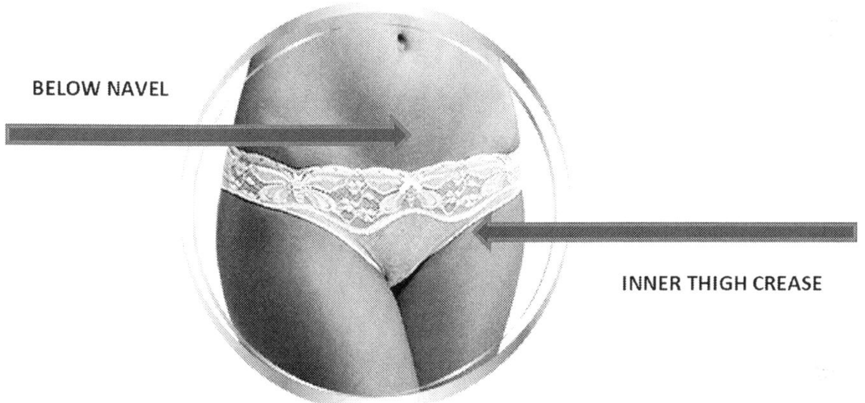

Vaginal Dryness

What about lubrication? It is vital for pleasurable sex. Unfortunately, the production of vaginal secretions subsides as we age.

The largest survey of US women, REVIVE (Real Women's Views of Treatment Options for Menopausal Vaginal Changes), included 3,046 women with symptoms of vaginal dryness and revealed the following:

85% of partnered women had some loss of intimacy

59% indicated their symptoms detracted from enjoyment of sex

47% of partnered women indicated it interfered with their relationship

Vaginal dryness occurs in many women, especially perimenopausal and postmenopausal women due to low estrogen levels. There is insufficient lubrication in the cervix which leads to inflammation and thinning of the vaginal walls, making sex uncomfortable, even painful. This is an easy fix. Some immediate things you can do include avoiding synthetic material in your underwear, not using scented and harsh soaps, and doing pelvic exercises like Kegels. You can also try vaginal massage (with or without your partner), leave more time for foreplay, and/or try a natural chemical free lubricant.

I was shocked to learn the ingredients in most lubricants on the market. Vaginas are lined with mucous membranes that secrete and absorb fluids faster than skin, as do the clitoris, vulva and urethra. Most lubricants contain chemicals that can damage vaginal tissues, and can increase the risk of bacterial vaginosis and sexually transmitted diseases such as herpes and chlamydia. These chemicals disrupt a woman's internal pH and beneficial microbes.

I switched years ago to organic coconut oil as a natural lubricant. It is easy to get at the grocery store, convenient to use, affordable, and it's antibacterial and antifungal. *Coconut oil will break down latex condoms, so if you are still in perimenopause, make sure to use a different contraceptive-still not responsible for any unintended pregnancies.* Other natural lubricants are pure aloe vera gel, olive oil, flaxseed oil, vitamin E oil, almond oil, or distilled water. You can add essential oils to the coconut oil and make your own lube, but never use essential oils undiluted on sensitive areas. Try adding some of the Vitality® ingestible oils for some edible fun. (Wink wink).

Should you have any kind of skin reaction to the homemade massage oil/lubricant, again, grab some plain coconut oil or other oil, not water, and apply to the affected area. It will help relieve whatever reaction you may have.

Sensation Massage Oil®

Having learned about the toxicity in most everyday products, and now knowing that your vagina is highly absorbable, it makes sense—unless you are going to make your own lubricant—to try Sensation® Massage Oil as an alternative. It is a combination of coconut, grapeseed oil, almond and olive oil combined with the essential oils Ylang Ylang, Geranium, Bergamot, Coriander and Jasmine. And it smells and feels luxurious. Start off the night using it to give him a back massage and end the night with a full body massage on you both. Take note of the different carrier oils in the Sensation Massage Oil® ingredients if you have any allergies.

Clary Sage

The natural lubricants are perfect for in the moment, but if you want to support natural production of lubrication for the vagina in general, use Clary Sage daily applied a couple of inches below the belly button a couple of times a day. As estrogen productions slows down, we start to dry up. Clary Sage is an oil that can support the hormonal system and in turn may help keep us moist.

Shutran®

I can't do a chapter on sex and the oils and not include Shutran®. It was created as cologne for men, but I'm telling you, in my experience it is a gift for a woman. Shutran® has a scent that makes you want to jump your partner's bones. It helps release inhibitions.

It helps support his performance and endurance. Although he can apply it ALL over, you can also apply it topically to your inner thigh for a VavaVoom evening. Some menopausal women have been in a relationship for a very long time with the same person. They need to get creative to keep things interesting. Shutran® was our game changer. It can be yours too.

More Favorites

Other favorite oils to get things rocking are Patchouli, Orange, and Geranium for me and Hong Kuai, Goldenrod and Idaho Blue Spruce for him and we've got the bedroom covered!

Do you feel better now knowing you aren't the only one having trouble between the sheets and that you now have real solutions? Check out these diffuser and lubricant recipes to get you back to feeling like the hottie you are.

#REALTIONSHIPGOALS FOOT MASSAGE

1. Start by rubbing your partner's feet slowly, applying gentle pressure, for a few minutes to release any tension. Some lotion or massage oil will help your fingers slide easier over their feet.
2. Move to the inside anklebone.
3. Make small, gentle circles in the groove below the anklebone. Rub the tips of your thumbs side to side across this sensitive area; make sure to go all the way around the ankle and toward the Achilles tendon too.

   This is the part of the foot that relates to the sex organs. Massaging it can relieve sexual tension and awaken things for both of you down under . Just go easy. The area can be quite sensitive.

I'M IN THE MOOD FOR LOVE

4 drops Ylang Ylang

2 drops Orange

2 drops Joy®

Diffuse in the bedroom.

SWEET & SPICY EDIBLE MASSAGE OIL

1 / 4 cup organic coconut oil

1 drop Cinnamon Bark Vitality®

1 drop Peppermint Vitality®

2 drops Orange Vitality®

2 drops Lemon Vitality®

Combine ingredients in a glass jar or glass container with a pump.

NOTES

Help! Fat Has Found Me And It Won't Let Go!

I've had many clients share the identical story as they entered their menopausal years: The weight just comes on and won't go away, even among traditionally fit women who haven't changed their eating or exercise habits. I know now, through my own experience, that their story is true. Within a few months of starting to skip my periods, I gained almost 15 unwelcomed pounds, and it's been a struggle to take them off. For a while it was lose a pound/gain two, lose 2 pounds/gain 1, getting me nowhere. My old methods of losing weight weren't working. My 80/20 rule of eating healthy 80% of the time and indulging the other 20% was failing me. I admit, I probably (OK, definitely) got a little lazy too and may have indulged a bit more and exercised a bit less. But I am someone who refuses to deprive myself, so I needed to figure out which elements in my diet needed tweaking. I knew my eating and exercise routines weren't up to snuff, but suddenly I was feeling tired, all sorts of blah, and unmotivated throughout the day. I realized my hormones must be playing a role in my weight gain, as they seemed to have taken over many areas of my life.

According to nutritionist, Mickey Harpaz, PhD, author of *Menopause Reset! Reverse Weight Gain, Speed Fat Loss, and Get Your Body Back in 3 Simple Steps*, "Women going through menopause can gain 8 to 15 pounds in the first two years if they aren't careful." Not great news for us. Bethany Barone Gibbs, PhD, an epidemiologist at the

University of Pittsburgh, conducted a 2012 study investigating the relationship between eating habits and weight gain in postmenopausal women. She concluded, "Your goal is to make small changes that you can maintain for the rest of your life." This is totally in line with my philosophy and what I have taught to clients in my nutrition, weight loss, and fitness practice for years. Like it or not, for many women the onset of menopause signals it's their time to change up old eating and exercise habits.

As we all know, change isn't easy, but we are likely to make better choices if we understand WHY maintaining a healthy weight is important during our perimenopausal and postmenopausal years. There's no denying I'd love to have a chiseled 20-something body, but mostly now I just want to feel good, look in the mirror and see a fit, strong, healthy me. Choosing the right foods and the appropriate exercises can make that goal achievable.

Here are 4 awesome reasons to shake things up a little:

1) Your body needs to detoxify from years of exposure to pesticides, chemicals and heavy metals.
2) Eating whole foods may reduce your food cravings and hot flashes.
3) Exercising increases our levels of youth HGH (human growth hormone), which preserves bone health and lean muscle mass and also helps to reduce stress.
4) Improved cardiovascular health prevents the #1 killer of women over 50: heart disease.

DETOXIFICATION

You're now aware that if you've lived for any period of time on this planet, you've been exposed to chemicals just from everyday living. When trying to manage weight in your 40's and beyond, a detox or cleanse of the body is a great place to start. There are many different detoxes and cleanses out there. Some may help rid your cells of the toxin overload they've been exposed to, allowing them to communicate better. Other detoxes help to release unwanted toxic buildup in your fat cells so that you can more easily shed unwanted pounds. Some help to reduce sugar cravings and reset the body so that it can better receive the good nutrition you are now going to feed it. Because you will continue to exist on Earth for many years and will be exposed to chemicals and other elements no matter how hard you try to avoid them, be aware that doing a detox isn't a one-time permanent fix. Dr. Mark Hyman, renowned physician and author of *The Blood Sugar Solution*, recommends a gentle detoxification one to two times a year.

5 Day Nutritive Cleanse®

I have done many different detoxes and cleanses over the year and have tried the Young Living 5 Day Nutritive Cleanse® a few times. It was gentle and relatively easy. It's a meal replacement in the form of a delicious shake three times a day, a couple of shots of Ningxia Red® juice daily, a digestive support supplement to take before eating, and optional snacks. When I completed the 5 Day Nutritive Cleanse®, my body felt clean, my mind felt clear, and my constant need for chocolate was gone.

Cleansing Trio®

The book *Inner Transformations with Essential Oils* by Drs. Leanne and David Deardeuff, D.C., provides cleansing protocols for overall well-being. The Deardeuffs recommend as a colon cleanse Young Living's Cleansing Trio®, which uses essential oil infused supplements. When essential oils are added to the supplements, it makes them more readily absorbed into the body and makes better use of the nutrients by softening the cell's thickened membranes caused by the toxic buildup.

Cleansing Oils

Did you know there are foods and essential oils that can help cleanse your body and help you reach and support a healthy weight? Many people already know to squeeze a fresh lemon into their water daily. Famous doctor and TV personality Dr. Mehmet Oz says that adding lemon to hot water is a great way to rev up your metabolism for the day and kick start your energy. As a substitute for an actual lemon, one can add a drop of Lemon Vitality® or Citrus Fresh Vitality® oil to their water. Using the oil makes on-the-go use easy. . . . I mean, what woman wants to carry lemons in her purse? I have had clients in a weight loss rut see the scale start to move again once they added Lemon Vitality® oil to their water a few times a day. Citrus Fresh Vitality® is a combination of five different citrus oils plus Spearmint Vitality® oil. The Spearmint Vitality® oil may help with healthy digestion. As you make other dietary changes, your body may need extra support to adjust and citrus oils can help.

Heavy Metal Cleansing

Toxic exposure to heavy metals such as cadmium and lead can be problematic during menopause. In an abstract in The Journal of the British Menopause Society, the authors report that about 90% of lead in the body is found in the bone. They state that there "is a significant release of bone lead after the menopause, in association with the acceleration of bone resorption. Thus, postmenopausal women may be at increased risk of adverse effects of lead. The lead released may cause neurological, kidney and gastrointestinal effects." Yikes! Sounds like an excellent reason to do a "heavy metal" cleanse. In another of Dr. Hyman's books, *Ultra Protection: The 6 Week Plan That Will Make You Healthy for Life*, Hyman advises to "add cilantro to meals, it removes heavy metals." The constituents found in Cilantro bind to the heavy metals which are then eliminated. Try making a fresh salsa with organic cilantro and Lime Vitality® oil for your next snack! Although there are differing opinions on whether essential oils can remove heavy metals from the body, it is agreed that certain essential oils can support the body's natural detoxification process.

Although other heavy metal cleansing is needed, some foods and essential oils may contribute to the removal of the heavy metals.

Increase Your Fiber

Another way to clean up your body is to increase your fiber intake. Increased fiber helps your body digest and eliminate easier and faster, but can result in more time on the toilet. Most people consume around 14 grams of fiber per day, even though the daily recommendation is 20 to 35 grams. According to www.cancer.net, it is much healthier for postmenopausal women to not reabsorb estrogen into their colon, as this lowers breast and uterine cancer risk. Increasing your daily fiber intake to 35 to 45 grams can slow down this reabsorption. Cruciferous vegetables including cauliflower, broccoli, kale and cabbage are good for moving the bowels. Stir fry style cooking is a quick, easy and inexpensive way to add these veggies to your diet. Grab a pan, heat up some coconut oil, throw in some of your favorite veggies including the cruciferous ones, and add some shellfish, chicken or tofu that has sat in a healthy, low sodium marinade. Use a toothpick to stir in one of the Vitality® herb oils such as Basil Vitality® or Rosemary Vitality® oils to taste (note that one drop of oils can pack a ton of flavor; see suggestions for cooking with oils below).

Flax seed is also high in fiber. If you're having hot flashes, try throwing some ground flax seeds into your smoothies or salads; it may just help reduce them. What a bonus! But remember, if you increase your fiber intake, you must also increase your water intake. A general rule of thumb is to drink at least half your weight in ounces of water each day (for example, if you weigh 160 pounds you should aim to drink 80 OUNCES of water daily).

Add the essential oil Digize Vitality® to your water. The fennel, anise and ginger in this oil may provide you with digestive support for the increased amount of fiber which your body may not be used to.

Another source of good fiber is Balance Complete Meal Replacement®, containing 11 grams of fiber from multiple sources of natural fiber. Its yummy, vanilla cream flavor is great to throw in smoothies or oatmeal for an added boost. But it also tastes great by itself in water and is part of the 5-day Nutritive Cleanse.

LESS SUGAR, MORE FRUITS AND VEGGIES

In the Australian longitudinal study on women's health, eating less sugar and drinking less alcohol reduced hot flashes and night sweats. The study also found that reducing caffeine intake can also have a similar effect. Unfortunately, menopause is a wakeup call to review those longstanding dependencies on coffee to stay awake and wine to fall asleep. If you have a spare tire around your waist that seems to have found a permanent home there, reducing or eliminating your sugar, alcohol and caffeine might be a good place to start. The hormone fluctuations we experience during menopause can affect our body's ability to maintain stable blood sugar levels, making sugar reduction vital to weight loss and maintenance.

Lean, Mean, Anti-Oxidant Fighting Machine

One way to achieve this at meals is to fill your plate with lots of veggies and some fruits first, before grabbing for the main course or other extras. This will naturally help you to eat more of the foods most beneficial to you and less of the foods that may not be in your best interest. Fruits and vegetables are generally high in fiber and will fill you up (plus we need the extra fiber anyway).

Fruits and vegetables are also high in antioxidants, which help combat the unwanted health impact from the pollution, plastics, processed foods, and other enemies found in our environment. I mentioned earlier Dr. Christiane Northup, who found that low antioxidant levels can also contribute to hot flashes. Drinking smoothies is an easy way to raise our antioxidant levels and to also get more plant-based foods into our bodies. Throw your favorite protein powder and fruits and vegetables into a blender, add some flax seed (if you have hot flashes and for extra fiber), a drop or two of an essential oil and some water or non-dairy milk and you're in business.

Since protein intake is important for women over 50 to help build and maintain muscle to stay fit and strong, adding protein powder to a smoothie, such as Pure Protein Complete Chocolate® with 25 grams of protein per serving, is an easy and healthy addition.

Maca

In my research on natural solutions for the issues I was experiencing, I also learned about raw maca powder, as well as gelatinized maca, for hormonal balance and supporting menopause and started throwing it into my smoothies. Maca powder is a yummy superfood, dried and ground from a Peruvian root vegetable that resembles a small turnip and contains a variety of beneficial nutrients including vitamins (vitamins A, B, C,

D and E), minerals (such as iron, magnesium, calcium, potassium, and iodine), fiber, amino acids and essential fatty acids. Maca powder has special properties that may create hormonal balance within the body, which is what can make it so effective in relieving menopausal symptoms. Gelatinized maca is maca root that's been lightly processed to remove the starch, making it easier to digest while still keeping most of the nutrients intact. In an article by Gustavo F. Gonzales in the journal, *Evidence-Based Complementary and Alternative Medicine,* he included numerous clinical studies on maca. Some of these studies have indicated that maca has a positive effect on energy levels and mood and can help to reduce anxiety and simultaneously increase libido. Wow! Who would've thought one could drink a smoothie and not only increase your antioxidant level, fiber and boost your protein intake, but also reduce hot flashes, feel horny, chill out and also satisfy an overwhelming craving for sugar by providing a healthy sugar fix? Sign me up!

Bye, Bye Sweet Tooth

There are countless low-sugar "foods" found at the market, which contain artificial sweeteners you should avoid at all costs. Read labels. DO YOUR OWN RESEARCH. These low-sugar alternatives can cause serious damage to our bodies. It is better to seek natural sugar sources such as small amounts of raw honey, 100% pure maple syrup or quality stevia.

Using essential oils can help take care of that annoying sweet tooth. Adding Slique Essence® oil to your water can get you past the mid-afternoon "I must have sugar NOW!" hump. It has three different citrus oils combined with Spearmint and Ocotea oils. Ocotea is related to the cinnamon plant. It has many wonderful properties that may help with maintaining a healthy weight, a healthy heart and desired blood sugar levels. Studies have shown that Ocotea may also help curb cravings and promote feelings of fullness. It creates a delicious blend which is specifically designed to support healthy weight management.

If you're looking for another low sugar, no caffeine afternoon pick-me-up or evening "mocktail," consider trying Ningxia Red® juice, mentioned earlier as a part of the 5-Day Nutritive Cleanse®. Ningxia Red® combines the Ningxia Wolfberry®, which is rated as having one of the highest antioxidant concentrations of all foods. The addition of plum, pomegranate and cherry, plus high-antioxidant aronia berry and blueberries, makes Ningxia Red® an excellent, delicious source of added protection from exposure to pollution, pesticides and plastics. Ningxia Red® juice is also infused with Orange, Lemon, Tangerine and Yuzu oil, which can be great for digestive support and overall wellness.

Ningxia Red® is a delicious option that may support healthy blood sugar levels. One to two, 2 ounce daily shots of Ningxia Red® and not only do you feel great, but because of the synergy of the different fruits, berries and oils you are, in a single ounce of juice, consuming , according to the antioxidant equivalent of 100 oranges or 814 blueberries or nearly 11 pounds of spinach. You couldn't eat that amount in one or even a dozen sittings! Many people will add oils like Copaiba Vitality® and Frankincense Vitality® to their Ningxia Red® for an extra boost of wellness. Others like to "party" by spiking their Ningxia Red® with oils such as Peppermint Vitality® or Thieves Vitality®, which produce a WOW effect as they go down.

I created this chart for a quick reference to foods that will benefit you the most during menopause. Take this list the next time you go shopping! Although eating in moderation is a necessity, it is equally important to eat foods that will bring the most benefit to your changing body's needs.

EAT MORE DURING MENOPAUSE	EAT LESS DURING MENOPAUSE
Dark, leafy green vegetables (Kale, Bok Choy)	Candies, cakes, brownies, including low sugar versions
Almonds	Alcohol
Walnuts	Milk
Apples	Bagels
Beans	Corn
Edamame	White or processed grains
Chickpeas	Potatoes
Sweet potatoes	Dried fruit
Pineapple	Bananas
Shellfish	Cereal
Avocado	Bread
Garlic	Cheese
Onion	Yogurt
Beets	Pizza
Blueberries	Hamburgers
Wild Salmon	Red meats
Tomatoes	Chicken
Cabbage	Coffee (caffeinated)
Eggs	Soda
Olive Oil	Spicy foods
Oranges	Hot soups
Broccoli	Warm beverages
Fermented Foods	Milk
Peppermint Tea	French Fries
Wild Salmon	Ice Cream
Cauliflower	Rice
Quinoa	Overly processed soy
Flax Seed	Vegetable Oil
Whole grain pasta	Fast Food
Almond, Coconut milk	Frozen Meals
Nut butters (almond, cashew)	Artificial Sweeteners

EXERCISE: A MUST AT MENOPAUSE ONSET

An increase in high intensity exercise can improve production of the Human Growth Hormone (HgH), the hormone associated with youthfulness and vitality. The level of this hormone declines as we age. A depletion of HgH levels results in a decrease in lean body mass, testosterone and estrogen production, along with a decline in bone density and immune function. Lower HgH levels also lead to an increase in fat surrounding our organs and can create sleep, vision and skin disturbances. Menopausal women are susceptible to all of these issues. In other words, the more HgH, the merrier you'll be.

One reason your weight loss may have stalled is from performing the wrong kinds of exercise to increase your HgH. Maybe you've always been a distance runner or a CrossFit junkie. But now nothing is budging no matter how long you run or how much weight you lift. Maybe in the past all you had to do to lose weight was jump on the elliptical machine while reading a magazine for an hour and the pounds simply melted away. Well guess what? The times they are a-changing. Exercises that create the best results for menopausal women are high intensity/short interval workouts mixed in with stretching and body/mind exercises. You can perform repeated sprints, interval training, weight training or circuit training to increase your HgH levels and maximize fat loss.

Releasing the Human Growth Hormone (HgH)

To create a release of HgH, you must first increase your body temperature. You need to kick things into high gear, go beyond your comfort zone and get out of breath. Exercise in short 10-30 second bursts of 90% to 100% maximum intensity effort. This might look like 30 seconds of jumping jacks or push-ups followed by a 15-second rest, repeated for 2 to 4 minutes. This cycle allows your body to experience a phenomenon called "oxygen debt." It is this oxygen debt that triggers the HgH release. Increase your intensity and endurance by rolling Raven® or Breathe Again® essential oil containing eucalyptus on your chest for added respiratory support. Research on eucalyptus shows that it "contains a number of compounds with antispasmodic, anti-harmful organism, expectorant, and decongestant properties," according to an article by Dr. Edward Group, DC, *"The Lung Cleansing Benefits of Eucalyptus."* If you are huffing and puffing from giving it your all, just pause, roll on the Breathe Again and get moving again! Of course listen to your body and stop if needed but if you 've got a drop more to give, roll away!

Don't stop when you feel the burn—it's a good sign! That burn is the key to revving up your metabolism and getting rid of that fat through the release of HgH. The Young Living® essential oil infused supplement Powergize® is perfect for anyone who wants to amp up their workouts with sustained energy, strength and focus. Oil-infused supplements such as Aminowise® can help support your muscles during and after exercise, and also help to fight fatigue and enhance your post-workout recovery. Stretching both before and after a workout is crucial to for keeping the body flexible and free of pain.

Bend And Balance

Speaking of flexible, both flexibility and balance become more important as we age. The wear and tear of life is showing up in the form of aches and pains and the inability to bounce back up from the floor easily. In addition, falling down becomes a real possibility to be feared. Adding Yoga and Pilates between these high intensity workouts will help you improve your ability to reach, bend and feel steady on your feet.

Pilates has the added benefit of strengthening your pelvic floor muscles, which are often shot from childbirth and aging. I've actually had Pilates clients claim their husbands thank ME for their improved sex life due to their wives' newfound deep muscle strength down below!

Yoga and Pilates are also great for stress relief. As we now know, increased stress causes increased cortisol production which leads to stubborn belly fat. Try diffusing essential oils such as Gathering® or Grounding® while doing these mindful exercises for added relaxation, grounding and release.

Building Strong Bones

One of the reasons exercise is so important is that it helps us maintain good bone health. The article "The Assessment of Fracture Risk" found in the *Journal of Bone and Joint Surgery* claims osteoporosis "affects up to 40% of postmenopausal women." This higher risk for osteoporosis puts us at greater risk for fractures and injuries from falls.

Bone quality is of upmost concern for menopausal women because we lose calcium due to osteoporosis. Lots of money has been poured into osteoporosis medications, but a report in the *Archives of Internal Medicine* links the use of these medicines to a higher risk of unusual fractures in the thighbone. Although studies have shown those drugs help prevent spine and hip fractures in the short term (3-4 years), there hasn't been much research to support their use long-term, yet women often remain on these medications for a long time. The FDA looked at 3 long-term studies to determine whether these drugs had any effect after 5 years. They found that the benefits lessened at 5 years, and those who took the medications for 6 years or more had more fractures than those who took a placebo drug.

In a special health report from Harvard Medical School, *Osteoporosis: A Guide to Prevention and Treatment*, the authors suggest taking care of your bones with an exercise routine that includes aerobics, strength training, balance and flexibility. Bones need stress to strengthen, and exercises such swimming and walking (which are often prescribed to women over 50) are not enough. Studies done by Sinaki (1989 & 2010) show that weight bearing exercises, along with exercises to strengthen balance and flexibility, can decrease bone degeneration as effectively as osteoporosis medications.

Body Weight/Small Equipment Exercise

You can increase your muscle mass through body weights, small weights and resistance exercises that reinforce everyday movement patterns. Body weight exercises including squats (not too deep though) help ease movements like bending down to pick up groceries. Other exercises where all you need are you and a mat are pushups, lunges, tricep dips, squats, planks and lots more. Small weights between two and five pounds, exercise bands, and kettlebells are great for weight bearing exercises at home. Grab some soup cans if that's all you have!

Agilease®

The Young Living supplement Agilease® works preventatively to support and improve joint and cartilage health. It can help relieve the normal aches and pains you may feel after a workout. Some of my favorite oils after a tough workout are Deep Relief® and Pan Away®. Both of these blends include Wintergreen, which is known for its ability to support joints and muscles so we can go about our daily activities. After I get out of the shower after exercising, I like to use the Orthosport Massage oil® to ease any remaining muscle tension from my workout. If I have time, an even better option is to combine a cup of Epsom salt, 1 cup of baking soda and 15 drops of Lavender oil and draw a bath and sprinkle.

Along with proper exercise, you definitely need the right amount of calcium to maintain proper bone health. The National Institute of Health recommends 1,200 mg of calcium daily. Although we often associate calcium with strong bones, we also need calcium for our muscle, nerve and cardiac function. In fact, the body prioritizes these areas over bones. Calcium levels can decrease due to an acidic diet from excessive amounts of animal products and sugars. Other calcium thieves include smoking, alcohol, stress, caffeine, and inflammation. Your body will actually take calcium from your bones and give it to the heart. The safest and most effective way to obtain and utilize calcium is through whole food nutrition. Many people think dairy when they think calcium, but dairy intake has some unhealthy side effects and many people do not tolerate it well. According to Dr. Hyman, "Dairy is one of the biggest triggers of hormonal imbalances because of all the hormones found naturally in milk and because of the hormones and antibiotics added to milk. In fact, dairy has over 60 hormones that can contribute to imbalances." Alternatively, some researchers believe that large amounts of dairy consumption may actually delay menopause. Choose non-dairy calcium sources such as seeds, some nuts, and leafy greens. Because there is a great deal of conflicting research about calcium supplements and menopause, I suggest that postmenopausal women get their calcium naturally from their diet and not from calcium supplements. But if you do choose to use a supplement, consider Young Living's SuperCal® Plus which contains calcium, magnesium and many other minerals and is infused with essential oils. It also contains Vitamin D which helps absorb the calcium. According to the National Osteoporosis Foundation, both Vitamin D and Calcium have been shown to support strong bones as we age.

HEART ATTACK

Heart disease in women has been on the rise. According to the American Heart Association, since 1984 women's deaths due to cardiovascular disease have exceeded those of males. Approximately 380,000 women per year have a heart attack. Twenty-six percent of women ages 45 and older who have had a heart attack will die within 12 months. Sixty-four percent of women who die suddenly will have experienced no previous symptoms. This is why it is vital we take care of ourselves and don't wait until tragedy strikes. Fortunately, most cardiovascular issues can be slowed or even reversed with some good old fashioned healthy eating and exercise that gets the heart pumping.

Fats should represent less than 20 percent of your daily menopause diet. You might need to experiment a bit. First, consider your fat source. We need more fats from avocados and olive oil and fewer saturated fats such as meat and dairy. My teenage daughter makes a quick and tasty guacamole with a couple of added drops of Lime Vitaity® essential oil.

Avoid buying "low fat" or "fat free" foods because they are usually loaded up with sugar so they taste good. Ningxia Red® juice is also great for supporting cardiovascular health.

Omegagize®

Omega-3 fatty acids (fish oil) help reduce LDL (bad) cholesterol and lower the risk of heart disease. Women who are at greater risk of heart disease after menopause may want to take a fish oil supplement, or simply increase the amount of fish they eat. The American Heart Association recommends eating at least two servings of fish per week. For vegetarians, Omega 3's can also come from walnuts and flaxseed. (There's that flaxseed again—seems like a must-have for the menopausal woman's kitchen!) One study found that taking EPA (one of the omega-3 fatty acids found in fish oil) as a supplement reduced the number, but not the severity, of hot flashes in menopausal women. Just one more excellent reason to take your Omegas. You can use a supplement such as Young Living's Omegagize® which, in addition to the needed fish oils, also includes Vitamin D3 and CoQ10 and essential oils that may support heart health as well as brain, eye, and joint health.

Stress Be Gone

Since we're on the subject of heart disease, let's discuss stress-related heart attacks. Coronary heart disease is more common in individuals subjected to chronic stress, according to the British Heart Foundation: "Constant stress has been linked to higher activity in an area of the brain linked to processing emotions, and an increased likelihood of developing heart and circulatory disease."

We have learned what stress can do to our bodies. The body creates cortisol when stressed out. This can increase our risk of cardiovascular problems, contribute to weight gain and cause fatigue. Cortistop® is an herbal supplement which is designed with DHEA, black cohosh, pregnenolone and essential oils to help women's bodies reduce cortisol levels that are elevated by everyday stressors. Young Living's supplements are infused with essential oils. When essential oils are added to herbal, vitamin or mineral supplements they help with the absorption of the nutrients and are more effective. Cortistop® can help reenergize you and may help you manage a healthy weight and heart.

Another amazing outlet for releasing stress and staying heart healthy—EXERCISE! Just one more reason to do it! But what about foods to reduce to stress? There are some good choices according to the Physician's Committee for Responsible Medicine. They recommend low fat, high-fiber, carbohydrate-rich meals with plenty of fruits and vegetables. "They soothe us without sapping out energy and give us the nutrients we need to boost our immune system." And make sure to avoid sugar and caffeine which many of us turn to when stressed, as they are often a temporary high from which you come crashing down.

There are so many components that go into living through these menopausal years, but a chemical-free body fueled by healthy, fresh foods and sustained with safe, effective exercise is the best foundation.

MELTING THE MENOPAUSE MIDDLE EXERCISE PROGRAM

Download a body weight exercise program designed specifically for the menopausal woman's needs at www.jilllebofsky.com. You will also find some demo videos of the exercises to assure you use proper form and safety while exercising.

HAPPY HORMONES SMOOTHIE

8 oz. of water or nondairy milk

Scoop of Balance Complete Vanilla Meal Replacement® (or a vanilla protein powder)

1/2 banana

1/2 cup of frozen cubed mango (or fresh—just add a few ice cubes)

1/4 cup frozen pineapple (optional)

1-2 cups of chopped spinach or kale

4 drops of Orange Vitality® essential oil

1 Tbs. ground flaxseed

1 Tbs. maca root powder (optional)

Toss ingredients into a blender and blend until smooth.

ROASTED RED PEPPER CARMELIZED CAULIFLOWER QUINOA SALAD

1 medium head cauliflower

1 Tbs. coconut oil

2 red peppers

1/2 cup uncooked quinoa (I like to use red)

1/2 cup water

1/2 cup vegetable broth (optional—can substitute with more water)

1 Tbs. ground flaxseed

1/4 cup minced cilantro

1/4 cup minced flat leaf parsley

(FOR THE DRESSING)

3 Tbs. olive oil

2 Tbs. lime juice (approx. juice of one lime)

4-5 drops of Lime Vitality® essential oil (or zest of a lime)

2 Tbs. raw honey

1/4 cup lightly toasted pepitas (raw pumpkin seeds)

Preheat oven to 425° F.

Cut cauliflower into bitesize florets.

Toss with 1 Tbs. coconut oil.

Place whole red peppers on a baking sheet.

Add cauliflower to baking sheet.

Roast, turning occasionally, until cauliflower is caramelized and peppers charred, approx. 25-35 minutes.

Remove from oven and let cool slightly. Remove the skin from the roasted red pepper and dice.

Rinse quinoa if not pre-rinsed and combine with water and veggie broth (or all water) in a medium pot. Bring to a boil, reduce to a simmer, and cook until water is almost fully absorbed, about 12-15 minutes. Remove from heat, cover and let sit until remaining water is absorbed, about 5 minutes. Stir in the flaxseed.

Combine quinoa, cauliflower, and roasted red pepper in a bowl.

Add cilantro and parsley to quinoa mixture.

To make dressing, combine olive oil, lime juice, Lime Vitality® oil and honey in a jar with liquid.

Shake until combined. Pour on salad and toss until combined.

Add toasted pumpkin seeds. Taste and add salt as desired.

Recipe adapted from Naturally Ella at www.naturallyella.com

NOTES

Is That ME In The Mirror?

I'm now at the age where I "get it" when people say things like "age is just a number" and "I still feel 20 inside." Truthfully, I loved my 20's, kid-free and travelling the country, but I neither expect nor want to look THAT young anymore. We should all feel grateful for the wonderful experiences that gave us the eye crinkles from smiling so much and the important moments that left "worry" lines on our foreheads, earned through years of parenting or striving to achieve in our jobs. We can't stop our faces from changing, but now we also know that we should have listened to Mom and used sunblock and moisturizer every day and possibly spared our skin. The best thing we can do now is to try and reverse or slow down the aging process or maintain and enhance our skin to better match our outer appearance to our inner age, to how we truly feel inside. A good place to start is with a plant- and mineral-based sunscreen. The last thing we want to do is spray or rub chemicals on our bodies that get quickly absorbed through our skin and then bake in the sun. Living in Florida, there is no escaping the sunshine (lucky me!). I make sure to use my Young Living Mineral Sunscreen Lotion® every day which contains zinc and essential oils like Carrot Seed, which has a natural SPF. I mix the sunscreen into my moisturizer. Easy peasy!

Changing levels of hormones, particularly estrogen, also affect our complexion and hair. Some of the most frequent complaints I hear when it comes to beauty include dry, wrinkled, sagging skin; hair thinning on heads but springing up in unwanted areas like the chin; and acne breakouts like we're 14 again. Collagen and elastin are the two major components that keep our skin youthful and smooth, but their production naturally diminishes as we age. Dr. Mickey Harpaz, mentioned previously for his book *Menopause Rest!* wrote on the website *Menopause Matters* that collagen production decreases by 30% within 5 years of menopause onset. Decreased estrogen levels accelerate collagen decline, causing our fine lines, wrinkles and sagging. Blood flow is also reduced due to estrogen playing a role in blood vessel maintenance. As we enter menopause, our skin's barrier (the outermost layer of skin) starts weakening and thinning and losing water, causing dry, scaly, flaky skin and scalps. The shift in balance between estrogen and testosterone levels causes pimples to pop up, especially on our chins and necks. The sweating at night or the hot flashes during the day can also contribute to our faces acting up. Not to mention decreased estrogen's contribution to thinning hair, which nearly all women experience by age 50.

There are a million products out there promoted as the "Fountain of Youth." According to the website Statista.com, in 2016, in the United States alone, the beauty and personal care industry generated approximately $84 billion dollars in revenue. The cosmetics industry has manipulated us into believing that youth is better, more attractive. Baloney! We have fallen for this false notion that as we age we become less desirable. Many people are willing to try any product if there's potential that their wrinkles will cease to exist or their stretch marks or cellulite will vanish. I get it, I too want to look my best, I want to look fresh and aglow, but I also want to embrace myself right where I am in life. Yes, this means preserving and enhancing the features I have, but not at the cost of my health. Many women are so blinded by society's version of beauty that they don't care or realize the physical costs they are paying with their health from all these toxic goops and chemical laden makeups.

This is your skin we are talking about. The largest organ in your body and one of the most absorbent. This is where your due diligence in researching commercial cures becomes so important. Don't waste your money on products that may get rid of a wrinkle or two yet at the same time contain a cancer causing ingredient. Essential oils and some other plant- based products can be just as effective, if not more effective and much more affordable.

Face Favorites

Some of my favorite essential oils for maintaining a smooth, perky appearance are Lavender, Frankincense, Myrrh, Manuka and Sandalwood. There are many homemade recipes for facial washes and moisturizers using unscented Castille soap and coconut oil and adding in the essential oils.

Orange Blossom Facial Wash®

If you want to address hormonal acne, try using Orange Blossom® facial wash with Orange Blossom, Rose and Lavender, Lemon, Patchouli® and Rosemary oil. Teens love it (I have a teenage daughter), and we women are now dealing with teenage skin issues. If you are looking for an everyday, lighter face soap, the ART Facial Cleaner® is good for daily use with oils including Frankincense, Myrrh, Sandalwood, Lemon and Melissa.

Wolfberry Eye Cream®

Those perfectly named crow's feet that have crept up around your eyes can be lessened naturally with Wolfberry Eye Cream®. We learned about the high antioxidant content in Ningxia Wolfberries® and the effect antioxidants can have in combating the aging process, including the impact on our skin. The combination of wolfberry seed oil and other carrier oils and the essential oils Lavender, Roman Chamomile and Geranium helps minimize fine lines and soothes tired eyes.

Sandalwood Moisture Cream®

Different skin types require different moisturizers, but most women with dry skin find great results with Sandalwood Moisture Cream®. It also has the Wolfberry seed oil and Sandalwood, Lavender, Myrrh and Rosemary essential oils. It's rejuvenating!

Boswellia Wrinkle Cream®

Many women also enjoy the Boswellia Wrinkle Cream®, with the power of Frankincense. It also contains MSM—a sulphur compound that supports collagen to improve their skin's firmness. And we need collagen support, for as we learned, we lose collagen as we age.

Mint Satin Facial Scrub®

Because our skin is constantly exposed, it is important to do a gentle scrub to clean out our pores from debris. The Mint Satin Facial Scrub®, used on your face twice a week, is gentle and cooling and your face just shines after applying it!

Sensation Hand & Body Lotion®

And let's not forget the rest of your body. You can make a nice sugar body scrub, infusing it with Peppermint, for a great morning start. Use hand and body lotion when you get out of the shower to keep your skin moist and supple. Might I suggest the Sensation

Hand & Body Lotion® after an evening shower, especially before a night of romance?

Makeup Makeover

After going through all the trouble of cleaning and moisturizing our face with these healthy, chemical-free, plant-based products, most of us will grab our foundation and blush and lip stick without thinking twice and put these chemical cosmetics all over our freshly preserved face, totally defeating the point! Do I need to remind you about parabens and their toxic friends? Many women after 50 aim for a more natural look, some foregoing makeup altogether. Some makeup can have the exact opposite effect we were hoping for and age us instead of enhancing the God-given beauty we have. It's time for more ingredient review and research. Your makeup should be free of lead, parabens, bismuth, dyes, parabens, and synthetic colorants. If you are looking for a totally chemical- free makeup that gives you a natural, fresh look, then Young Living's Savvy Minerals® makeup line was made for you. Although women of all ages love the Savvy Minerals® look, I think the natural look and glow this makeup gives is perfect for women over 50 to bring out their sexy, confident selves!

Hair, There, Everywhere!

How many of you have noticed more hair in the bottom of the shower or coming out in your brush? Are there areas of your hair where it's obviously not as thick as it used to be, leaving you balding as your hair thins from hormonal deficiencies? The good news is that if hair thinning is due to menopause, the situation is reversible. There are some ways you can support hair strength and growth. Proper nutrition is one, especially finding a good source of iron. Essential oils such as Cedarwood and Rosemary have also been found to support healthy hair, and you can easily make sprays or can even add a few drops to your shampoo. Use a plant-based shampoo such as Copaiba Vanilla® or Lavender Mint Shampoo®. The infusion of essential oils enhances the benefits to your hair.

And what about those unwanted chin hairs that are growing at a rate that's hard to keep up with? One old tried and true solution for that—TWEEZERS! With a pluck pluck here and a pluck pluck there . . . Some other natural suggestions from Karen Reed, managing editor of *Positive Health Wellness*, are facial waxing using honey or molasses, an egg white mask that hardens and removes the hairs when you peel it off, and a papaya/turmeric scrub.

Papaya contains an enzyme that breaks down the hair follicles, preventing them from growing more hairs. Adding turmeric into the mix makes the papaya more effective. The compounds in tumeric will help kill off the hairs, preventing their regrowth. There is a link to some of Karen's recipes at the end of this chapter.

For those of you who remember the 80's, there was a Billy Crystal skit on *Saturday Night Live,* whose character always said the popular tagline, "It's better to look good than to feel good." Well, we are older and wiser and we want both.

SMOOTH AS SILK MOISTURIZER

Coconut or jojoba oil as a carrier oil

8 drops each of Lavender, Frankincense, Myrrh, Manuka, Patchouli essential oils (You can use just Frankincense and Lavender)

Put essential oils in a 10 ml roll-on and mix together.

Fill the rest of the way with coconut oil. Roll on face after your wash and toner.

OR

Place 2-3 Tbs. of coconut oil in glass container and mix in oils and keep in a jar in the bathroom.

END OF THE DAY MAKEUP REMOVER PADS

4 oz. jar

2 Tbs. Coconut oil as a carrier oil

1 tsp. Unscented liquid castille soap

Distilled water

1/2 tsp. Vitamin E Organic cotton facial round pads

4 drops of Lavender essential oil

Place cotton rounds in a small mason jar, squeezing in as many as you can.

Combine the coconut oil, castille soap and Vitamin E.

Pour mixture over cotton pads and press down on them so they evenly get absorbed.

Pour water over the pads until wet. Place the lid on the jar and shake it up.

Can also be used as everyday facial cleansing pads.

LUXURIOUS LOCKS HAIR REGROWTH & STRENGTHENER

2 oz. jojoba oil or coconut oil as a carrier oil

5 drops Rosemary

5 drops Cedarwood

10 drops of Lavender

2 drops of Peppermint

Combine ingredients in a bowl or bottle with a pump and gently massage into the scalp, preferably before bed so it can work overnight. Use a Young Living® shampoo for daily use.

MORNING START BODY SCRUB

4 oz. mason jar

1/3 cup organic white or brown sugar

2 Tbs. coconut oil

10 drops of Peppermint essential oil

Combine the sugar and coconut oil.

Stir in the Peppermint oil.

Add to the Mason jar.

Adjust drops to scent to your taste.

NOT BY THE HAIRS ON MY CHINNY CHIN CHIN

Egg White Mask & Papaya Tumeric Scrub recipes mentioned above can be found at: bit.ly/naturallyremovehair

NOTES

The Many Moods of Menopause

Moody? Who, *me?* Never. It's everyone else who's moody, and *they're* the ones affecting *my* mood, right? Well, all right, maybe it *is* me—sometimes. Of all the changes in my body as I begin perimenopause, I definitely feel changes to my emotional health the most. Can you relate? One minute you are fine, and the next minute you are either snapping at somebody or wanting to cry. Many emotions surface at this life stage. Many women report feeling depressed and anxious. Others feel lonely, isolated, and bored now that their days no longer revolve around their kids' schedules. Still others go from calmness to a complete rage in a nanosecond. Women's concerns about their health or their spouse's health take over their thoughts as new aches and pains occur. Then there are financial worries: How would we take care of ourselves should something major happen to our partner? And what about divorce? Not something we want to think about, but we covered "gray divorce" in Chapter 4, and how divorce rates are rising among 45- to 55-year olds according to Pew Research Center, leaving women to deal with many new responsibilities previously handled by their exes. Major life changes can be overwhelming and strip away the person we REALLY are. Add in the hormonal rollercoaster, and some women cannot deal. They may turn to alcohol to take the edge off, which also contributes to weight gain. The evening glass of wine turns into three to four drinks or more a day just to cope. Some women turn to dangerous prescription pills to get through the day and sleep through the night.

One of my closest friends is 75 years old. When I shared with her how out of sorts I felt due to my perimenopausal issues, she said, "this is the time in your life when all the stuff you've shoved deep down for years comes up for you to deal with." According to a study from the University of Wisconsin-Oshkosh, between 1850 and 1900, many women were sent to insane asylums for mental health conditions relating to their normal bodily functions. The researchers found "suppressed menstruation" (aka menopause) to be a common reason for admittance. And only 120 years ago, husbands could have their wives imprisoned for using foul language and being too emotional. Let's just say I'm happy to be living in *these* times! Although who could blame my poor husband, living with a hormonal wife and two hormonal teens? The kids have their own "attitude adjuster" essential oil blend, but I have found that using Progessence Plus® and Clary Sage consistently, one drop of each twice a day (I'm using them for my hot flashes too – that's two benefits!) has helped keep me much more even keeled.

Some of the things we physically experience at this time in our lives actually have emotional roots. Hot flashes may be a manifestation of your feelings. Many women experience hot flashes when they are angry, especially if they don't have an outlet for their anger. Vicki Noble, author of *Shakti Woman: Feeling Our Fire, Healing Our World* suggests, "Hot flashes are the body's way of naturally cleansing what it no longer needs." One of the best ways to overcome negative feelings is through keeping a journal. Find a quiet space, put some essential oils in your diffuser and write those feelings right out of your head. You can diffuse oils such as Peace & Calming® and Joy® to create a serene and uplifted mood.

Emotional Release

Essential oils may also help us release buried emotions from old trauma or deeply seeded beliefs we may not even realize we hold about ourselves. We need to face our demons or negative emotions head on, and essential oils are an easy and natural way to uplift our mood, let go of hurt and anger and step into the best versions of ourselves. The essential oil blend Release®, placed between the lower ribs and stomach toward the right side of the body, over the liver (an organ thought to store anger) is a great place to start. Other essential oil blends such as Forgiveness®, Acceptance®, and Hope® can be powerful allies to help you deal with difficult feelings once and for all. In the book, *Releasing Emotional Patterns with Essential Oils,* author Carolyn Mein, DC, recommends the appropriate oils to use for specific emotional issues, where on your body to put them and includes a positive affirmation statement to say aloud to help reprogram and change negative belief patterns. You'll find some examples in the next chapter. I *highly* recommend this book if you're struggling emotionally. You can also seek out a certified Aroma Freedom Technique® practitioner, who can provide another way to use essential oils to achieve emotional balance.

Putting Yourself First

Women of menopausal age have spent decades putting their own needs last. We've been loyal daughters, wives, mothers and employees, but many of us have lost a piece of our "self" along the way. Our kids are older and need us less, or perhaps they're already "grown and flown" away. The empty nest can contribute to loneliness and all the normal life changes that may be occurring, such as downsizing a house or retiring, can cause angst, even depression for some. But . . . this is the time in our lives we've been waiting for! We now have TIME, well-earned time for putting *ourselves* first, yet we aren't feeling good. We need to practice self-care, which is so important to our mental state. We can't give in to these emotions and curl up and hide under a blanket on our couches. We are vibrant, beautiful, needed, worthy women! What things do you enjoy doing? Who do you enjoy doing them with? What do you like to do to relax and release stress? Work on a craft project. Go for a walk in the woods. Catch up on the phone with a good friend for lunch. Pursue greater adventures: travel, bucket list items, or go out and start making a difference in the world. This is a time for self-discovery and trying new things.

Ideas For Relaxing & Enjoying Life & Rediscovering You

- Spend time with your hand in soil tending your garden. Try growing your own garden.
- Sit quietly by water (ocean, river pond) and just listen.
- Grab a magazine or book (the real thing—not a screen) and read.
- Meet up with a favorite friend you haven't seen in awhile.
- Pamper yourself. Get a massage, organic facial or mani/pedi.
- Shut off all devices for an hour every day and do something creative.
- Start every day by journaling or visualizing your day exactly as you'd like it to unfold.
- Play with your pet. Find a new trail to walk. Look for a dog park and meet new people.

Adding essential oils into your "me time" routine will elevate your mood to a different level. Consider getting a monthly Raindrop Technique® massage from a trained therapist, which utilizes a combination of many different essential oils for total body relaxation. You will soon be in La La Land. How about a super simple meditation practice to start your day using Frankincense? Bring the mountains to YOU while you inhale the scent of Pine oil or Northern Lights Black Spruce®. Or relax with a glass of wine and your favorite music in the background while diffusing Harmony® or Stress Away® oil.

Counting Sheep

Another major issue many women face during menopause is sleep disturbances. These can include anything from insomnia to waking up in the middle of the night to anxiety riddled nightmares. Night sweats or frequent bathroom runs are just part of the problem. Depression and anxiety can each contribute to sleep issues, or can be triggered by lack of sleep. All the hormonal changes, including a decrease in production of estrogen and progesterone, have an effect as well.

Michael J. Breus, PhD, a clinical psychologist with a specialty in sleep disorders says that "one of estrogen's functions in a woman's body is to regulate other hormones and neurotransmitters, including several that affect mood." These "mood-shaping hormones" also "play direct roles in regulating sleep-wake cycles".

Progesterone is known for its calming, relaxing benefits. It makes sense if there is a decline in progesterone production that there might be increased restlessness. In addition to using the oils for specific issues related to mood, the oils can support a good night's sleep. Diffusing a combination of Lavender and Cedarwood is a great way to drift off. Add in some Peace & Calming® and you will be out for the night!

We don't need to let our irrational hormonal thoughts get the best of us. We don't have to run and hide away from the world. We don't need to walk around like zombies with dark circles under our eyes. Try using essential oils that specifically support hormonal balance. At the same time, incorporate other essential oils into an activity that lifts your mood and decreases your stress level and supports sleep. These mental pick-me-ups are vital for your emotional well-being during menopause.

IF MAMA AIN'T HAPPY, NO ONE IS HAPPY

3 drops of Citrus Fresh®

2 drops of Orange

1 drop of Lime

Diffuse the following oils and smile.

"ALL IS WELL" ROLL-ON

10 drops Joy®

8 drops Stress Away®

8 drops Peppermint

10 drops Clary Sage (optional)

In a 10 ml roll-on, add the essential oils and fill the rest with coconut oil or any carrier oil.

DIFFUSE THE SITUATION BRACELET

Stretchy beading elastic cord Lava beads

Other plastic or non-porous beads that you want to customize your bracelet (find them at Walmart, Michael's or Amazon)

1 to 2 drops of your favorite essential oil

String the beads and tie off bracelet to fit your wrist. Put a drop or 2 of your favorite oil on the lava beads.

The scent should last a few days.

NOTES

Reinventing YOU!

I had a friend tell me the other day that, in her words, she "squashed her dreams long ago" and "doesn't know how to dream." This seriously hit me in the gut. How many other women over 50 feel this way? How can they change this feeling ASAP? If it's been awhile since you thought about what you REALLY want your life to look like, then this may take some time, but it's so worth it. Rediscovering YOU is a crucial piece of the menopausal puzzle.

Building Your Dream

What did you want to be when you were a little girl? I wanted to be an Olympic ice skater like my idol Dorothy Hamill. Had her haircut and everything. Envisioning your future helps lay the groundwork for it to happen. You have to think it before it becomes a reality. But many women have put their dreams on hold for so many years that they don't know where to start. Women who have been out of the workforce for years raising children may feel like they don't have the skills needed today to succeed. So wrong! Don't discount the leadership skills you practiced in chairing PTA meetings or the conflict management skills you developed while navigating your teenagers' dramas or your ability to do three things at once without breaking a sweat. You've been an artist, a chef, a banker, a doctor, a teacher, a coach and everything in between. Essential oils can help pull that dream out of you and make it a reality. Oils like the Envision®, Build Your Dream® and Highest Potential® blends were created with that purpose in mind, to awaken and inspire your dreams and goals. Roll them on or diffuse them—or better yet, do both—then grab a piece of paper, find a quiet spot and start writing down things you enjoy doing, things you are good at doing, things or people that inspire you, and things that fulfill you then sit with that list awhile and see what ideas pops up for you. Maybe you decide to start your own photography business—you've been taking pictures of your family for years and everyone always tells you how good you are. Maybe you decide to write the book you've had brewing inside you for years. Maybe you decide to sell everything and travel the world. The exact dream doesn't matter, all that matters is that you DREAM!

But a dream is simply an unanswered wish if not followed with action. To make change you have to take action, inspired action. Roll on some Inspiration® oil, take a big breath in and take the first step. This combination of 10 oils includes Cedarwood, Sandalwood and Frankincense. These oils were used during biblical times, but also by Native Americans for hundreds of years, for prayer, meditation and spiritual connection.

Fighting The Negativity

Motivational speaker Jim Rohn claims that "You are the average of the five people you spend the most time with." Choose wisely. Take a close look at your life and the lives of those around you. Are these people feeding your inner fire to BE, to DO and to HAVE more, or are they trying to extinguish it? People tend to remain within their comfort zone. And when you decide to rock the boat, to try something new and step out of your complacency, some people won't like it. They may even feel threatened by it. But that's their problem. I suggest that if you MUST keep some of the negative Nellie's in your life, put a drop of White Angelica® on your shoulders next time you see them as protective "angel wings" to lift you above their lackluster energy. You don't need THEIR negativity as you build YOUR positivity and create your future.

Into The Future® is a powerful essential oil blend which keeps you focused on where you want to go without getting distracted!

We have plenty of negative voices in our own heads telling us we aren't good enough or capable. These oils will help you face what holds you back from going after everything you want in life, get out of your own way and take the first step.

Gratitude®

I think the best place to start reinventing yourself as you create this second half of your life's journey is to be grateful for all that you have now in your life and for all the people and things that taught you important life lessons along the way. And yes (of course!), there's an essential oil called Gratitude® for that and it includes spiritually elevating oils such as, Balsam Fir and Myrrh. In the article, *In Praise of Gratitude,* published by Harvard Medical School, the authors define gratitude as a "thankful appreciation for what an individual receives, tangible or intangible." The article reviewed many different studies on gratitude and found that most "support an association between gratitude and an individual's well-being." Start a practice of beginning and ending every day with a drop of Gratitude® in your palm, and after a few deep inhales think of at least three things you are grateful for in that moment to feel an inner shift in your thoughts and feelings.

Just Believe

You have always been everyone's cheerleader—now you need to be your own! That starts with belief in you. When you use essential oils such as Believe® and Abundance® regularly, you feel not only a shift toward positivity inside of you, but an amazing change occurs on the outside. At least twice a day I will put a drop of each in my palm and inhale a few times and I swear miracles happen. My phone starts ringing with opportunities, or I'll receive a random email about something I was just thinking about and needed help with. An inspired idea will come to me. Money will just show up out of the blue. I can't explain how it works; I only know I've experienced it over and over again and am a believer.

Transformation®

Then there is Transformation® essential oil, also with Sandalwood, Balsam Fir and Frankincense. What better time for this oil than during one of the most significant metamorphoses of your life? This blend of 8 different oils was made for the menopausal woman whose body and life is in transition. This blend was created to help release old beliefs and solidify new ones. Try diffusing this oil while you sleep. For me, it is the one time I'm quiet, my brain and body resting, so my unconscious mind can go to work.

I Am Woman, And You're Gonna Hear Me Roar

Our beliefs are merely repeated thinking patterns we've developed since childhood. Some serve us, some limit us. A disconnect is often created between what we want and what we feel we deserve. Positive affirmations combined with essential oils can be powerful and used for spiritual and personal growth to close this gap. Positive affirmations are statements of truth which one aspires to absorb into their life. They aren't just a wish on a star. According to self-help expert Louise Hay, "An affirmation opens the door. It's a beginning point on a path to change." Affirmations are how we tell the subconscious "I'm ready."

Affirmations are best said aloud and even better spoken in front of a mirror so you are truly facing yourself. It may feel strange and uncomfortable at first but stick with it.

Diffuse the oils mentioned in this chapter or inhale the scent of a few drops on your hands as you say your affirmation. "I AM" statements are good ones, such as "I AM in charge of my health and happiness," or "I AM on my perfect path." Stand over your diffuser, close your eyes, take four to five deep breaths, look up, stand up straight, relax your shoulders and loudly and with conviction repeat your affirmation a few times. Now, if you have teenagers in the house they may make fun of you, so you can say it a little quieter but with the same power! Even if you don't feel the words at first and feel completely ridiculous (I know I did), say them anyway. Fake it 'til you make it I say! Do this every night before sleeping and first thing when you wake up to start your day and you will become a force to be reckoned with!

We are strong. We are WOMAN! Ready to take on the world!

UNSTOPPABLE! PERFUME

10 drops of Believe®

10 drops of Inspiration®

10 drops of Highest Potential®

In a 10 ml roll-on, add the oils and fill the rest with coconut oil or a carrier oil.

IMAGINE THE FUTURE DIFFUSER BLEND

3 drops of Envision®

3 drops of Awaken®

1 drop of Pine

Add essential oils to the diffuser.

ABUNDANT LIFE ROLL-ON

10 Drops of Gratitude®

20 drops of Abundance®

Coconut oil or other carrier oil

In a 10 ml roll-on, add the oils and fill the rest with coconut oil or a carrier oil.

NOTES

And In the End...

How do you feel now that you have knowledge and solutions? I hope you feel empowered to face your perimenopausal and postmenopausal changes, using essential oils as part of your support team. Those words don't sound as scary now, do they? Can you envision yourself in your best physical and emotional health? Can you see you and your partner enjoying a renewed honeymoon period?

Menopause doesn't need to feel like a personal prison, with you at the mercy of the hot flash and belly fat guards imposing their will on you. Essential oils combined with other healthy lifestyle choices can release us from these old notions of menopause as a disorder to be endured quietly and alone, a stigma, an ending. We women have and always will overcome whatever life throws at us. A menopausal woman armed with knowledge of how her body and mind works as it moves through these new changes is not enough. She needs practical solutions and those are what I have shared. Now it is up to you to take action. Continue to research and learn more about using essential oils and other natural means to enhance your change of life. Pay close attention to what your body wants and needs and give it that. Experiment, track your results and most important, SHARE with other women your experiences loudly and proudly so we can demolish the image of the crazy old lady and replace it with the best version of ourselves.

MY FAVORITE YOUNG LIVING PRODUCTS THAT MAY SUPPORT A HEALTHY MENOPAUSE

HOT FLASHES/NIGHT SWEATS

Clary Sage

Fennel

Geranium

Lady Sclareol®

Lavender

Lemon

Peace & Calming®

Peppermint

Prenolone Plus Body Cream®

Progessence Plus®

Roman Chamomile

Sclaressence®

LIBIDO/VAGINAL DRYNESS

Bergamot

Clary Sage

Geranium

Goldenrod

Hong Kuai

Idaho Blue Spruce

Jasmine

Joy®

Lady Sclareol®

Neroli

Orange

Patchouli

Prenolone Plus Body Cream®

Progessence Plus®

Rose

Sandalwood

Sclaressence®

Sensation®

Sensation Massage Oil®

Sensation Hand & Body Lotion®

Shutran®

Ylang Ylang

DETOXIFICATION/WEIGHT MANAGEMENT/HEART HEALTHY

5 Day Nutritive Cleanse®

Agilease®

Aminowise®

Balance Complete Meal Replacement®

Basil Vitality®

Breathe Again Roll-On®

Citrus Fresh Vitality®

Cleansing Trio®

Copaiba

Copaiba Vitality®

Cortistop®

Deep Relief Roll-On®

Digize Vitality®

Frankincense Vitality®

Ginger Vitality®

Lemon Vitality®

Lime Vitality®

Ningxia Red®

Ningxia Wolfberries®

Ocotea

Omegagize®

Oregano Vitality®

Orthosport Massage Oil®

Panaway®

Peppermint Vitality®

Powergize®

Pure Protein Complete®

Raven®

Slique Essence®

Spearmint Vitality®

Super Cal®

Tangerine Vitality®

Thieves Fruit & Veggie Wash®

Thieves Vitality®

Wintergreen

BEAUTY

ART Skin Care System®

Boswellia Wrinkle Cream®

Carrot Seed

Cedarwood

Copaiba Vanilla Shampoo & Conditioner®

Frankincense

Geranium

Lavender

Manuka

Myrrh

Ningxia Red®

Orange Blossom Face Wash®

Patchouli

Progessence Plus®

Rosemary

Sandalwood

Sandalwood Moisture Cream®

Mint Satin Facial Scrub®

Savvy Minerals Makeup®

Sensation Hand & Body Lotion®

MOOD/STRESS/SLEEP

Aroma Freedom Technique®

Acceptance®

Cedarwood

Citrus Fresh®

Clary Sage

Cortistop®

Forgiveness®

Frankincense

Gratitude®

Harmony®

Hope®

Joy®

Lady Sclareol®

Lavender

Lemon

Lime

Northern Lights Black Spruce®

Orange

Peace & Calming®

Peppermint

Pine

Progessence Plus®

Raindrop Massage®

Release®

Roman Chamomile

Rose

Sclaressence®

Stress Away®

Ylang Ylang

EMPOWER

Abundance®

Awaken®

Balsam Fir Believe®

Build Your Dream®

Cedarwood

Clarity®

Envision®

Frankincense

Gathering®

Highest Potential®

Myrrh

Northern Lights Black Spruce®

Pine

Sandalwood

Transformation®

White Angelica®

OTHER

Thieves Household Cleaner®

Thieves Laundry Soap®

Thieves Dish Soap®

Works Cited

3rd Age Certification®/ Burrell Education/ www.burrelleducation.com

Aldercreutz, H., and W. Mazur. "Phyto-Oestrogens and Western Diseases." *Ann Med,* 29 Apr. 1997, pp. 95–129., www.ncbi.nlm.nih.gov/pubmed/9187225.

"American Lung Association®." *American Lung Association,* www.lung.org/

Aroma Freedom Technique®/Aroma Freedom International/ https://aroma-freedom.myshopify.com/

Bloom, Linda, and Charlie Bloom. "The Epidemic of Gray Divorces." *Psychology Today,* Sussex Publishers, 2 Apr. 2012, www.psychologytoday.com/us/blog/stronger-the-broken-places/201204/the-epidemic-gray-divorces.

British Heart Foundation, www.bhf.org.uk/heart-matters-magazine/news/behind-the- headlines/stress-and-heart-disease

Calcium Fact Sheet for Consumers, ods.od.nih.gov/pdf/factsheets/Calcium-Consumer.pdf.

"Cancer.Net." *Cancer.Net,* www.cancer.net/.

Choi, et al. "Effects of Inhalation of Essential Oil of Citrus Aurantium L. Var. Amara on Menopausal Symptoms, Stress, and Estrogen in Postmenopausal Women: A Randomized Controlled Trial." *Evidence-Based Complementary and Alternative Medicine,* Hindawi, 12 June 2014, www.hindawi.com/journals/ecam/2014/796518/.

Deardeuff D.C., David and Leanne. *Inner Transformations Using Essential Oils: Powerful Cleansing Protocols for Increased Energy and Better Health,* 2006.

Environmental Working Group, www.ewg.org

Franchomme, P., et al. *L'aromathérapie Exactement.* Roger Jollois Editeur, 1991.

Gibbs, Bethany Barone, et al. "Effect of Improved Fitness beyond Weight Loss on Cardiovascular Risk Factors in Individuals with Type 2 Diabetes in the Look AHEAD Study." *European Journal of Preventive Cardiology,* U.S. National Library of Medicine, 25 Sept. 2012, www.ncbi.nlm.nih.gov/pmc/articles/PMC3812302/.

Gittleman, Ann Louise. *Before the Change: Taking Charge of Your Perimenopause.* HarperCollins Publishers, 2017.

Gonzalez, Gustavo. *Evidence-Based Complementary and Alternative Medicine - An Open Access Journal,* www.hindawi.com/journals/ecam/.

Gottfried, Sara. *The Hormone Cure Reclaim Balance, Sleep, and Sex Drive; Lose Weight; Feel Focused, Vital, and Energized Naturally with the Gottfried Protocol.* Scribner, 2014.

Group, Edward. "The Lung Cleansing Benefits of Eucalyptus." *Global Healing Center,* 14 Oct. 2015, www.globalhealingcenter.com/natural-health/lung-cleansing-benefits-of- eucalyptus/.

Halcon, Linda, University of Minnesota, Taking Charge of Your Health & Wellbeing, *How Do Essential Oils Work?* www.takingcharge.csh.umn.edu

Harpaz, Mickey, and Robert Wolff. *Menopause Reset!: Reverse Weight Gain, Speed Fat Loss, and Get Your Body Back in 3 Simple Steps.* Rodale, 2011.

Harpaz, Mickey. *Menopause Matters,* www.menopausematters.co.uk/.

Harvard Health Publishing. "In Praise of Gratitude – Harvard Health." *Harvard Health Blog,* www.health.harvard.edu/newsletter_article/in-praise-of-gratitude.

Hay, Louise. "The Power of Affirmations." *The Power of Affirmations,* 23 Aug. 2017, www.louisehay.com/the-power-of-affirmations/.

Higley, C., Higley, A., & Leatham, P. (1998). Aromatherapy A-Z. Hay House

Hudson , Tori. "Discovering the Health Benefits of Maca." *Women in Balance Institute,* 26 Oct. 2012, womeninbalance.org/2012/10/26/discovering-the-health-benefits-of-maca/.

Hyman, Mark, and Mark Liponis. *Ultraprevention: the 6-Week Plan That Will Make You Healthy for Life.* Simon & Schuster, 2005.

Hyman, Mark. *The Blood Sugar Solution: the Bestselling Programme for Preventing Diabetes, Losing Weight, and Feeling Great.* Yellow Kite, 2016.

"Introduction to Menopause." *Johns Hopkins Medicine Health Library,* www.hopkinsmedicine.org/healthlibrary/conditions/adult/gynecological_health/introduc tion_to_menopause_85,P01535.

J., Jing. "Top 10 Xenoestrogens, the Primary Cause of Estrogen Dominance." *Top 10 Xenoestrogens, the Primary Cause of Estrogen Dominance,* 13 Jan. 2018, www.cycleharmony.com/remedies/hormone-imbalance/top-10-xenoestrogens-the- primary-cause-of-estrogen-dominance.

Keller, Helen, *The World I Live In,* New York The Century Co, 1910

Kingsberg, S A, et al. "Vulvar and Vaginal Atrophy in Postmenopausal Women: Findings from the REVIVE (REal Women's VIews of Treatment Options for Menopausal Vaginal ChangEs) Survey." *The Journal of Sexual Medicine.,* U.S. National Library of Medicine, 16 May 2013, www.ncbi.nlm.nih.gov/pubmed/23679050.

Lark, Susan M., and Kimberly Day. *Dr. Susan Lark's Hormone Revolution: Yes, You Can Naturally Restore & Balance Your Own Hormones.* Portola Press, 2008.

LaRue, Amy. "Xenoestrogens: What Are They, How to Avoid Them." *Women in Balance Institute,* 26 Oct. 2017, womeninbalance.org/2012/10/26/xenoestrogens-what-are-they- how-to-avoid-them/.

Lee, Christina, et al. "Australian Longitudinal Study on Women's Health." *OUP Academic,* Oxford University Press, 13 May 2005, academic.oup.com/ije/article/34/5/987/645885.

"Mayo Clinic." *Mayo Clinic,* Mayo Foundation for Medical Education and Research, www.mayoclinic.org/.

Mein, Carolyn L., and Richard Alan. *Releasing Emotional Patterns with Essential Oils.* VisionWare Press, 2017.

The Merriam-Webster Dictionary. Merriam-Webster, 2005.

National Osteoporosis Foundation®, *National Osteoporosis Foundation,* www.nof.org

Neville, Andrew. "Sweating Through The Sheets? The Adrenal Connection To Menopause." *www.healing.org,* 9 Mar. 2016, www.healing.org/symptoms/menopausal-symptoms/.

Noble, Vicki. *Shakti Woman: Feeling Our Fire, Healing Our World: the New Female Shamanism.* HarperSanFrancisco, 1991.

Northrup, Christiane. *The Wisdom of Menopause.* Judy Piatkus, 2001.

"Office of Dietary Supplements - Calcium." *NIH Office of Dietary Supplements,* U.S. Department of Health and Human Services, 2 Mar. 2017, ods.od.nih.gov/factsheets/Calcium-HealthProfessional/.

O'Reilly, Jessica. *The New Sex Bible: the Complete Guide to Sexual Love.* Quiver, an Imprint of Quarto Publishing Group USA Inc., 2017.

Physicians Committee for Responsible Medicine®, *How To Eat Right To Reduce Stress,* www.pcrm.org

Pouba, Katherine, and Ashley Tianen. "Lunacy in the 19th Century: Women's Admission to Asylums in United States of America." *Lunacy in the 19th Century: Women's Admission to Asylums in United States of America.,* University of Wisconsin Oshkosh, May 2006, www.minds.wisconsin.edu/handle/1793/6687.

Purser, Dan. www.natural-aromatherapy-benefits.com/support-files/progessence-plus- serum-dr-dan-purser-faq.pdf.

Reed, Karen. "9 Ways To Get Rid Of Facial Hair Naturally (That Actually Work)." *Positive Health Wellness,* 14 Mar. 2018, www.positivehealthwellness.com/beauty-aging/9-ways-to- get-rid-of-facial-hair-naturally-that-actually-work/.

Shifren, JL, and S. Hanfling. "Changes in Hormone Levels." *Sexuality in Midlife and Beyond: Special Health Report*, Harvard Health Publications, 2010, www.menopause.org/for- women/sexual-health-menopause-online/changes-at-midlife/changes-in-hormone-levels.

Shutes, Jade. *National Association for Holistic Aromatherapy*, naha.org/explore-aromatherapy/about-aromatherapy/what-are-essential-oils.

Sinaki, M, et al. "Efficacy of Nonloading Exercises in Prevention of Vertebral Bone Loss in Postmenopausal Women: a Controlled Trial." *Mayo Clinic Proceedings.*, U.S. National Library of Medicine, July 1989, www.ncbi.nlm.nih.gov/pubmed/2671517.

Sinaki, M, et al. "The Role of Exercise in the Treatment of Osteoporosis." *Current Osteoporosis Reports.*, U.S. National Library of Medicine, Sept. 2010, www.ncbi.nlm.nih.gov/pubmed/20574788.

Skin Care, Annmarie. "What's the Difference Between Collagen and Elastin?" *Annmarie Skin Care*, Annmarie Skin Care, 26 Mar. 2018, www.annmariegianni.com/whats-difference- collagen-elastin/.

"Skin Deep® Cosmetics Database." *Environmental Working Group*, www.ewg.org/skindeep

Smith, Mark S. "Doctor, Just What Is a Hot Flash?" *ObGyn.net*, 7 Oct. 2011, www.obgyn.net/hysterectomy/doctor-just-what-hot-flash.

Staff, Niha. "Integrative Health Blog." *Estrogen Dominance Doesn't Mean What You Think*, 5 Mar. 2012, info.nihadc.com/integrative-health-blog/bid/53256/estrogen-dominance-doesn-t-mean-what-you-think.

Stepler, Renee. "Led by Baby Boomers, Divorce Rates Climb for America's 50+ Population." *Pew Research Center,* 9 Mar. 2017, www.pewresearch.org/fact-tank/2017/03/09/led-by-baby-boomers-divorce-rates-climb-for-americas-50-population/.

Sunita, P., and S.P. Pattanayak. "Phytoestrogens in Post Menopausal Indications: A Theoretical Perspective." *Pharmacognosy Reviews,* Jan. 2011, pp. 41–47.

"Symptoms of Menopause and Sleep - The Sleep Doctor." *Your Guide to Better Sleep,* 29 Jan. 2018, www.thesleepdoctor.com/2018/01/09/symptoms-of-menopause.

Talbott, Shawn M. The Cortisol Connection: *Why Stress Makes You Fat and Ruins Your Health-and What You Can Do about It.* Hunter House, 2007.

Think Dirty Inc.® *"Think Dirty App",* www.thinkdirtyapp.com/.

Unnanuntana, A, et al. "The Assessment of Fracture Risk." *The Journal of Bone and Joint Surgery. American Volume.,* U.S. National Library of Medicine, Mar. 2010, www.ncbi.nlm.nih.gov/pubmed/20194335.

U.S. EPA. National Human Adipose Tissue Survey (NHATS). U.S. Environmental Protection Agency, Washington, D.C., 747-R-94-001,1994.

Vahter, M, et al. "Toxic Metals and the Menopause." *The Journal of the British Menopause Society.,* U.S. National Library of Medicine, June 2004, www.ncbi.nlm.nih.gov/pubmed/15207026.

Watson, Stephanie. "Thigh Fractures Linked to Osteoporosis Drugs; Long-Term Use Questioned." *Harvard Health Blog,* 21 May 2012, www.health.harvard.edu/blog/thigh- fractures-linked-to-osteoporosis-drugs-long-term-use-questioned-201205214737.

*Young Living Raindrop Technique®/Young Living/*www.youngliving.com/raindrop

*Young Living Seed to Seal®/Young Living/*www.seedtoseal.com

About Me

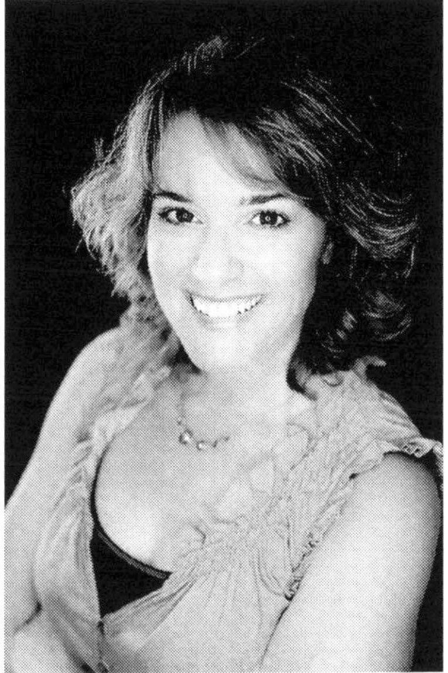

Jill Lebofsky just celebrated her 20th wedding anniversary with her college sweetheart. She is navigating the rough waters of parenting two teens and gets her doggie love from her Flat-coated Retriever, Ollie.

She is a Jill of all trades, following her passions and then teaching others what she's learned.

Jill started out as a Speech-Language Pathologist, helping adults regain the ability to talk, think and swallow safely after having a stroke, fighting cancer or living with Alzheimer's disease. But she soon realized preventative health care was where she could make a true difference. With small lifestyle changes, Jill knew people could avoid the problems she was seeing people suffer from unnecessarily.

She became a Weight Watchers leader after the birth of her second child, leading classes weekly at local meeting rooms and in corporate settings. This was the start of Jill's journey toward helping individuals shift their mindset about their relationships with food, themselves and others and teaching people how to eat healthy and incorporate movement into their lives.

In 2008 Jill became a Certified Pilates Instructor and ran her women only Pilates/TRX® studio Healthy U until 2016. In 2012 she was trained by The Institute for Integrative Nutrition as a Certified Health Coach and has created and facilitated many individual coaching sessions and group programs for hundreds of women and men over the years.

She has also received numerous specialty certifications to address the needs of women's wellness, including Breast Cancer Exercise Specialist® and the 3rd Age Woman® certification focused on eating, exercise and self-care for the perimenopausal years and beyond.

Jill was introduced to Young Living Essential Oils® in May of 2014 and has been sharing her oily love and knowledge ever since.

Jill is the author of 2 other e-books, "What to Eat When Your Plate Is Full" and "Scentsible Snacking".

STAY CONNECTED

Join our Facebook Private Group Page

"The Right Side of 45"

http://bit.ly/therightsideof45

Follow Jill on Instagram:

@therightsideof45

Check out Jill's website at:

www.jilllebofsky.com

OILY HELP HERE

Remember all oils aren't created equal and when using oils for a healthy menopause quality is vital. **To learn more about or purchase Young Living Essential Oils** speak with the person who introduced you to this book. Found me on your own and need help?

Message me at **jill.lebofsky@yahoo.com** to get connected.

BOOK JILL TO SPEAK AT YOUR NEXT EVENT!

Jill loves to educate and entertain whether it is on the big stage, small local gatherings or online. Go to www.jilllebofsky.com and check out some of the **topics available** for your group and connect for pricing and scheduling.

Made in the USA
Lexington, KY
12 November 2019

56919016R00066